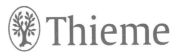

Ischemic Stroke Management: Medical, Interventional and Surgical Management

Alejandro M. Spiotta, MD, FAANS
Professor of Neurosurgery and Neuroendovascular Surgery
Program Director, Neurosurgery Residency
Director, Neuroendovascular Surgery
Medical University of South Carolina
Charleston, South Carolina

Roberto Crosa, MD
Chief of Endovascular Neurosurgery
Centro Endovascular Neurológico
Medica Uruguaya
Montevideo, Uruguay

46 illustrations

Thieme
New York • Stuttgart • Delhi • Rio de Janeiro

Library of Congress Cataloging-in-Publication Data

Library of Congress Control Number: 2019943242

Thieme Publishers New York
333 Seventh Avenue, New York, NY 10001 USA
+1 800 782 3488, customerservice@thieme.com

Thieme Publishers Stuttgart
Rüdigerstrasse 14, 70469 Stuttgart, Germany
+49 [0]711 8931 421, customerservice@thieme.de

Thieme Publishers Delhi
A-12, Second Floor, Sector-2, Noida-201301
Uttar Pradesh, India
+91 120 45 566 00, customerservice@thieme.in

Thieme Revinter Publicações Ltda.
Rua do Matoso, 170 – Tijuca
Rio de Janeiro RJ 20270-135 - Brasil
+55 21 2563-9702
www.thiemerevinter.com.br

Cover design: Thieme Publishing Group
Typesetting by Thomson Digital, India

Printed in the United States of America by
King Printing Co., Inc.   5 4 3 2 1

ISBN 978-1-62623-908-1

Also available as an e-book:
eISBN 978-1-62623-909-1

Important note: Medicine is an ever-changing science undergoing continual development. Research and clinical experience are continually expanding our knowledge, in particular our knowledge of proper treatment and drug therapy. Insofar as this book mentions any dosage or application, readers may rest assured that the authors, editors, and publishers have made every effort to ensure that such references are in accordance with **the state of knowledge at the time of production of the book.**

Nevertheless, this does not involve, imply, or express any guarantee or responsibility on the part of the publishers in respect to any dosage instructions and forms of applications stated in the book. **Every user is requested to examine carefully** the manufacturers' leaflets accompanying each drug and to check, if necessary in consultation with a physician or specialist, whether the dosage schedules mentioned therein or the contraindications stated by the manufacturers differ from the statements made in the present book. Such examination is particularly important with drugs that are either rarely used or have been newly released on the market. Every dosage schedule or every form of application used is entirely at the user's own risk and responsibility. The authors and publishers request every user to report to the publishers any discrepancies or inaccuracies noticed. If errors in this work are found after publication, errata will be posted at www.thieme.com on the product description page.

Some of the product names, patents, and registered designs referred to in this book are in fact registered trademarks or proprietary names even though specific reference to this fact is not always made in the text. Therefore, the appearance of a name without designation as proprietary is not to be construed as a representation by the publisher that it is in the public domain.

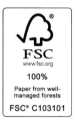

Contents

Preface

From the start, the purpose of this book was to try sharing our experience with other colleagues, the experience of so many years dedicated to this subject.

The present century has brought the most considerably advances in the study and treatment of this disease, which now, accounts for millions of deaths every year. Any improvement regarding mortality or quality of life for the survivors of this tragedy, will change the health system around the world in a relevant way, not only because this disease itself is devastating, but also on account of it being one of the leading consumers of resources. As far as imaging and treatment are concerned, we have witnessed a change in the paradigm: interpretation of stroke is more active and always implies the possibility of trying to revert it. Unfortunately, these paradigm changes are not detected with the same sensitivity in the whole range of medical and non-medical professionals, a situation that also arises in several other diseases. Neither are advances harmonically adopted worldwide, thus widening the gap between developed and developing countries. It is therefore our duty to embody in this book what we understand will help to improve and update among colleagues and medical students in the understanding of one of the most devastating and mortal diseases in the world.

To share a book with these characteristics with colleagues and friends that live and work so far away, is also a means to eliminate those frontiers and unite in a common project.

I consider many of the authors to be leading professionals in their specialties, and I can highly recommend reading their contributions.

The main characteristic of this book is that it does not discuss the experience of one center or of one technician. Perhaps that makes it more applicable to the environment of the reader. The authors of this book experience different daily realities, from South America to Europe, from North American to Asia. We have tried to unite our viewers about a subject, always using the best available scientific evidence.

There is no doubt that evidence presented from so many angles has changed forever the passive approach to this disease that prevailed not so long ago, namely on arrival all that was done was taking basic care of the patient and hope for the least possible damage. In terms of study and treatment, where there was almost nothing a few decades ago, we now have a wide range of possibilities that have made us change out approach to stroke, because perspectives have changed. All of the first-level evidence that has reaches the scientific community originates in countless colleagues and investigators that, although not contributing directly to this book, are a fundamental part of it because we have improved as specialists on account of their invaluable efforts.

Stroke has a particular trait that makes its awareness even more relevant for all the members of the health system. This trait is the intimate relation between the time elapses since the index event and the access to treatment. It is therefore basic that all, from the family physician to the neurosurgeon, should acquire due knowledge of one of the most frequent and invalidating diseases in the societies where they live and work.

However, this huge body of work in the field of neuroscience will be of little use if the different health systems do not adapt their protocols. It is useless to know the techniques for mechanical thrombectomy or the last advances in perfusion techniques if one cannot count on a system that previously prioritizes the patient and eliminates all obstacles in any system, if they prevent a timely treatment that could revert the course of such a devastating disease.

That is why this book is also intended to operate on an institutional level, because institutions play an essential and indispensable role in health policies in all countries.

The benefits of official action have been seen in several countries where the subject of stroke was treated as a problem of the state and great modifications in health planning were undertaken: mortality decreased and naturally, quality of life for the survivors improved.

Finally, I want to thank all of those who participated in this endeavor, writing with such a strict scientific approach and with such affection for those who deserve a better response from us....the patients with ischemic stroke.

Alejandro M. Spiotta, MD, FAANS
Roberto Crosa, MD

Contributors

Charles M. Andrews, MD
Associate Professor
Department of Emergency Medicine
Department of Neurosurgery
Medical University of South Carolina
Charleston, South Carolina

Carlos Batista, MD
Resident
Department of Neurology
Hospital de Clínicas de Porto Alegre
Porto Alegre, Brazil

Christopher Ludtka Beng, MD
Department of Neurosurgery
Helsinki University Hospital
Helsinki, Finland

Ana Canale, MD
Medical Coordinator, Staff Member
Intensive Care Unit
Hospital Pasteur, ASSE (Public Hospital)
Montevideo, Uruguay

Leonardo Augusto Carbonera, MD
Department of Neurology
Hospital Moinhos de Vento
Porto Alegre, Brazil

Carlos Castaño, MD, PhD
Doctor of Medicine and Surgery, Interventional
    Neuroradiologist and Neurosurgeon
Chief of Interventional Neuroradiology Unit
University Hospital Germans Trias i Pujol
Barcelona, Spain

Joham Choque-Velasquez, MD
Department of Neurosurgery
Helsinki University Hospital
Helsinki, Finland

Roberto Crosa, MD
Chief of Endovascular Neurosurgery
Centro Endovascular Neurológico
Medica Uruguaya
Montevideo, Uruguay

Ana Claudia de Souza, MSc, RN
Hospital Moinhos de Vento
Porto Alegre, Brazil

Adam A. Dmytriw, MD, MPH, MSc
Neuroradiology & Neurosurgical Services
Toronto Western Hospital, University of Toronto
Toronto Ontario, Canada
Beth Israel Deaconess Medical Center, Harvard
    Medical School
Boston, Massachusetts

David M. French, MD, FACEP, FAEMS
Associate Professor and Prehospital Director
Department of Emergency Medicine
Medical University of South Carolina
Charleston, South Carolina

Felix Göhre, MD
Department of Neurosciences
HUS Neurocenter
Helsinki, Finland

Pedro Grille, MD
Associate Professor
Intensive Care Unit
Hospital de Clínicas, UdelaR
Montevideo, Uruguay

Juha Hernesniemi, MD
Professor and Chairman
Juha Hernesniemi International Center for
    Neurosurgery
Henan Provincial People's Hospital
Zhengzhou, China

Christopher Alan Hilditch, BSc, MBBCh, FRCR
Consultant Neuroradiologist
Department of Neuroradiology
Salford Royal NHS Foundation Trust
Salford
Greater Manchester, United Kingdom

Behnam Rezai Jahromi, MB
Department of Neurosurgery
Helsinki University Hospital
Helsinki, Finland

Akitsugu Kawashima, MD, PhD
Chief
Department of Neurosurgery
Yachiyo Medical Center
Tokyo Women's Medical University
Chiba, Japan

Danil A. Kozyrev, MD
Department of Neurosurgery
Helsinki University Hospital
Helsinki, Finland
Department of Paediatric Neurology and
    Neurosurgery
North-western State Medical University
St. Petersburg, Russia

Dustin P. LeBlanc, MD
Assistant Professor
Department of Emergency Medicine
Medical University of South Carolina
Charleston, South Carolina

Sheila Cristina Ouriques Martins, MD, PhD
Professor of Neurology
Universidade Federal do Rio Grande do Sul, Hospital
    de Clínicas de Porto Alegre, Brazilian Stroke
    Network
Porto Alegre, RS, Brazil

Patrick Nicholson, MB BCh BAO, FFR (RCSI)
Clinical Fellow in Diagnostic and Interventional
    Neuroradiology
Division of Neuroradiology, Joint Department of
    Medical Imaging
Toronto Western Hospital
Toronto, Ontario, Canada

Vitor Mendes Pereira, MSc, MD
Professor
Department of Medical Imaging
Toronto Western Hospital
Toronto, Ontario, Canada

Nicolás Sgarbi, MD
Medicine Doctor, Diagnostic Neuroradiologist
Diagnostic MRI Department
MUCAM
Montevideo, Uruguay

Alejandro M. Spiotta, MD, FAANS
Professor of Neurosurgery and Neuroendovascular
    Surgery
Program Director, Neurosurgery Residency
Director, Neuroendovascular Surgery
Medical University of South Carolina
Charleston, South Carolina

Osmar Telis, MD
Department of Radiology
Hospital de Clínicas
Montevideo, Uruguay

Aquilla S. Turk, DO
Director of Neurointerventional Surgery Section
Associate Professor
Departments of Radiology and Neurosurgery
Medical University of South Carolina
Charleston, South Carolina

Paul M. Vespa, MD
Assistant Dean of Critical Care Medicine, Gary L.
    Brinderson Family Chair in Neurocritical Care,
    Professor of Neurology and Neurosurgery
Department Neurology and Neurosurgery
David Geffen School of Medicine at UCLA
Los Angeles, California

Joseph R. Whiteley, DO
Associate Professor
Department of Anesthesia & Perioperative Medicine
Medical University of South Carolina
Charleston, South Carolina

1 Stroke Epidemiology

Roberto Crosa, and Osmar Telis

Abstract

Stroke is one of the leading causes of morbidity and mortality among adults. More than 5 million people a year die of stroke around the world. It is difficult to evaluate incidence, prevalence and mortality on account of differences in registration. Most strokes are ischemic. Women have a higher incidence with a higher lifetime risk. Although the incidence in the high-income countries seems to be decreasing, the total burden of disease has not changed, and in fact may increase in the future, partly on account of an aging population. Transient ischemic attacks often precede stroke. Recurrent stroke is especially frequent after lobar hematoma. Secondary prevention and etiologic treatment have lowered somewhat the incidence of recurrent stroke. Mortality is substantial, both short-term and long-term, but a precise assessment is impossible due to surprising regional variations that are probably due to differences in reporting and registering. Global mortality tends to decrease, probably as a consequence of improved care. Non-modifiable risk factors include age, male sex, African ancestry, family history of stroke and genetic factors. Large vessel disease and cardioembolic stroke associate more frequently in women younger than 65. Modifiable risk factors, which account for 90% of stroke risk, are: hypertension (a major risk), diabetes (across all ages and ethnicities), arrhythmias (particularly if associated to AF and female sex), smoking, chronic kidney disease, oral estrogen therapy, sleep apnea. On consideration of the above, it becomes evident that stroke prevention requires a lifestyle change. Primary care physicians and health policies should cooperate to this end. Only a joint effort can decrease this pandemic significantly.

Keywords: stroke pandemic, ischemic stroke, hypertension, smoking, oral estrogen therapy, lifestyle change

1.1 Introduction

Stroke is one of the leading causes of morbidity and mortality in adults, with an increasing burden of disease in the adult and aging population. Worldwide, an estimated 16 million people per year suffer a stroke, leading to 5.7 million deaths.[1]

These results might be underestimated because of limitations in registry data and healthcare reporting in different countries or lack of access to healthcare in developing countries. Moreover, different studies might have slightly different results because of sample bias, making extrapolations difficult. It very likely that the true burden of disease is much higher, especially in developing countries, hence the need for better records, improved diagnostic algorithms, and faster access to optimum treatment, which are dealt with in other chapters.

Knowledge of the epidemiology of this worldwide pandemic is fundamental for public health policy, prevention strategy development and assessment of effective interventions. In this chapter, we review the current global findings of stroke epidemiology, its trends and associated risk factors.

Stroke epidemiology can be studied in two different ways, descriptive and analytical. Descriptive epidemiology tells us the frequency of the disease, and its changes through time, space and among different populations.[1] On the other hand, analytical epidemiology allows us to identify risk factors for stroke, and predictors of morbidity and mortality.[1] Both are necessary to effectively prevent and treat this disease.

1.2 Descriptive Epidemiology

The main indicators used in stroke descriptive epidemiology are prevalence, incidence, and mortality.

Incidence is the number of new cases in a specific population in a fixed period. This is a dynamic measurement, which can change between different periods of time, places, seasons, and can be affected by our efforts to fight against the specific disease.[1] It is expressed as a function of cases per person-time, and most often as cases per person-years, for a specific population.[1]

Prevalence is defined as the number of people with stroke at a specific moment of time, and represents the total burden at said moment. Prevalence can also be estimated over a period, integrating the incidence, as new cases during the study period, and the length of the disease. The higher the incidence and the longer the duration, the higher the prevalence in each period.[1]

Mortality rates represent the number of deaths in a fixed population over a period. In stroke epidemiology, both overall mortality and cause-specific mortality (deaths related directly to stroke) are used,[1] which may make interpretations difficult.

1.2.1 Stroke Prevalence

The worldwide prevalence in 2013 was an estimated 25.7 million, with approximately 10.3 million people having a first stroke in that year.[2] Most were ischemic in nature, and about 30% occurred in those younger than 65 years of age.[3] Due to the problems with reporting in different health systems and countries, it is likely that these findings are an underestimation of the real prevalence of stroke. There are, however, large sample studies available, mainly from developed countries, that provide essential information in this area.

Even though some findings suggest that age-adjusted mortality rates for ischemic and hemorrhagic stroke decreased between 1990 and 2013, the total number of strokes, related deaths and disability- adjusted life- years lost, increased.[4] In our opinion, it is very likely that this trend continues today, given the increase in life expectancy in recent years and that stroke prevalence increases with age.[4] Supporting this fact are findings from studies arising from the Behavioral Risk Factor Surveillance System (BRFSS) in the US, which shows that between 2006 to 2010, overall self-reported stroke prevalence did not change.[5]

Furthermore, in a US study of general population without prior diagnosis of stroke or TIA involving 18462 participants, the presence of least one neurologic symptom in those over 45 years old was 17.8%.[6] These findings strongly suggest that the true prevalence of stroke is even higher than estimated, with many undiagnosed or unreported events. These were more frequent in African Americans, those with lower education and income, and those with poor perceived health status,[6] which represent the more vulnerable populations in that country. Limitations in access to healthcare may also play a role in this population segment.

Finally, following worldwide trends, the prevalence of stroke in the US is expected to increase by 20.5% by 2030, compared to 2012.[7] In addition, prevalence of stroke survivors in the ageing population is expected to increase,[8] which will represent an increased challenge to healthcare systems and society as a whole. An optimization of prevention strategies and effective treatments will likely mitigate this expected increase, and might even prove predictions wrong. It is our responsibility as healthcare professionals to advocate for these changes to take place.

1.2.2 Stroke Incidence

Obtaining a global incidence statistic for stroke is a complex endeavor. The actual incidence varies greatly among different geographical regions, populations, and even across time.[1]

Worldwide, in 2010, there were an estimated 11.6 million ischemic strokes and 5.3 million hemorrhagic strokes, with increased incidence in low and middle-income countries.[9] This represents an incidence estimate of 258/100,000 people-year.[10] Between 1990 and 2010 the incidence of ischemic stroke fell by 13% in high income countries, but not in low or middle-income ones.[9] Furthermore, the incidence of hemorrhagic stroke decreased by 19% in high income countries, but increased by 22% in the rest with a higher burden on those 75 years old or younger.[9]

While socioeconomic status and an aging population clearly play a role, we believe that this also reflects the commitment of different countries to prevention and treatment of stroke, and to challenges in global healthcare, which must be addressed in following years to revert this situation.

The worldwide variations in incidence are far reaching across different populations, ranging from 130 to 410/100000 person-years.[1] There are also variations according to stroke subtypes, with the incidence of hemorrhagic stroke being significantly higher in Asian countries than in the Western world. This has been linked to a higher prevalence of hypertension in these populations, although other factors cannot be ruled out.[1]

In the US, about 795 000 people per year experience a new or recurrent stroke, of which approximately 610 000 are first attacks.[4] Of these, 87% are ischemic, 10% are ICH, and the remainder 3% are SAH strokes.[4]

Stroke incidence seems to be higher in those of African descent, with a lower incidence of cerebral infarction in women under 75, irrespective of ethnicity.[4] Among those aged 75 or older, African American women showed a higher incidence of cerebral infarction than men of the same ethnicity, while no difference was observed between white men and women aged 75 to 84.[4]

Women seem to have a higher incidence of stroke than men with a higher lifetime risk than men.[11] In the Framingham heart study, the lifetime risk was about 20% for women between 55 and 75 years of age, while it was approximately 15% for men of the same group. This seems to be at the expense of an increased incidence in older age groups and longer life span, since age adjusted incidence is lower for females in middle age or younger.[4]

Findings from both the BASIC Project between 2000 and 2010, the Framingham Heart Study, and Medicare recipients in the US show a reduction in incidence of global stroke over time[4] consistent with global findings of decreased incidence in high income countries.[12] Although incidence seems to be decreasing, the total burden of the disease has not changed, and is likely to increase,[1] especially with an aging population[12] and the increased prevalence of risk factors,[13] which we will discuss later in this chapter.

1.2.3 Transient Ischemic Attacks (TIA)

The knowledge of TIA epidemiology has a relevant role in stroke planning and prevention, since it is known that approximately 15% of all strokes are heralded by a TIA.[14] This means that appropriate evaluation, treatment and secondary prevention are mandatory for these patients. Failure to do so exposes them to potentially severe and life-threatening complications, and worsens their prognosis. In the US, it is estimated that that the prevalence of TIA was 2.3% overall, and increased with age. The real number is likely higher though, due to the same caveats of stroke research.[15]

A patient with a TIA is at a significant risk of short term complications, both neurologic and cardiovascular, and has an increased mortality risk. In one study of 1707 TIA patients evaluated in the emergency department in a northern California hospital, 5% had a stroke in the first 48 hours and 11% presented with stroke during the following 3 months. Risk factors for progression to stroke were age over 60 years old, diabetes, and duration over 10 minutes.[16]

Meta-analyses of cohorts of patients with TIA have shown that the risk of stroke in the first 48 hours is between 3% to 10%, and is 9% to 17% for the first three months.[17,18] Stroke risk at 10 years is approximately 19%.[4] Furthermore, the Oxford Vascular Study has shown that TIAs are a significant predictor of disability at 5 years.[19]

1.2.4 Recurrent Stroke

Recurrent stroke is a major complication in stroke survivors, with a major increase in morbidity and mortality. Several studies have assessed its prevalence and incidence, with results up to 18% recurrence rate at 4 years.[4]

Actual recurrence rates vary among different studies. A study in Northern Sweden, which followed 6700 patients who survived an ischemic stroke or had an intracranial hemorrhage between 1995 and 2008, showed that in this population recurrence rates were 6% at 1 year, 16% at year 5, and 25% at year 10 [20]. Another study which followed 10399 patients with a primary stroke in 2002 in the US, showed rates of 1.8% at 1 month, 5% at 6 months, 8% at 1 year, and 18.1% at 4 years.[21]

Recurrence rates vary according to etiology, stroke subtypes, and between studies. For hemorrhagic stroke, recurrence rates have been estimated at 2.4% per year, with a fourfold increase for lobar hematoma.[1] Most recurrences after both hemorrhagic and ischemic stroke are ischemic.[20] For ischemic strokes, rates were higher for those caused by large artery disease followed by small vessel disease and stroke of cardioembolic origin.[4] Also, a larger number of risk factors present is associated with higher recurrence rates.[4] Both diabetes and age at stroke are risk factors associated with increased risk of recurrence,[20] although all comorbidities play a role.

With minor variations, these findings are consistent across multiple studies in multiple populations of first world countries.[4]

In recent years, a decline in recurrence rates has been observed, probably due to better secondary prevention and etiologic treatment.[22,23] This should only strengthen our focus to improve on primary prevention, effective timely treatments and follow up, to reduce stroke's burden and improve outcomes.

1.2.5 Mortality

A recent report on global stroke statistics by Thrift et al[12] surveying all countries associated to the WHO has revealed an astonishing lack of accurate and recent data in over half of them, which makes evaluating true mortality difficult. This report also highlights significant differences between high income countries and low-middle income ones, where mortality adjusted by age seems to be higher, despite being probably underreported.

Mortality in stroke is substantial, both short-term and long-term. It varies significantly according to stroke subtype, being significantly higher for hemorrhagic subtypes in most studies, especially within the first month.[4] Further variances are observed across different populations, where age-adjusted mortality ranges from 41/100 000 people-years in Nigeria to 316/100 000 person-years in urban Dar-es-Salaam (Tanzania).[12] This large variation in mortality probably responds not only to intrinsic factors of each population, but also to differences in registry keeping and reporting between different countries. These large differences cast doubt on the actual available information. Another unexpected factor is the large difference between incidence and mortality rates in some low and middle-income countries, which are not concordant. There is probably a need for international organizations to directly take representative samples in different healthcare-challenged countries in order to properly assess stroke statistics.

The Atherosclerosis Risk in Communities Study (ARIC) study, which involved US patients from 4 different cities for a period of 24 years, showed a cumulative global mortality after index stroke of 10.5% at 1 month, 21.2% at 1 year, 39.8% at 5 years, and 58.4% at the end of follow up.[4] In the aforementioned Swedish study, a combined endpoint of recurrence and death was 28% at 5 years, and 45% at 10 years.[20] Furthermore, In the US, in 2014, stroke ranked 5th among leading causes of death, with a rate of 36.5/10000. These findings show the importance of secondary prevention and the dreadful long-term outcome a significant number of patients have after stroke.

Global trends suggest a decrease in mortality over the last 30 years of around 25%-30%.[4] This decline in mortality was more noteworthy in those over 65 years old, compared to younger age groups, although some studies show conflicting results in this regard.[24,25] Although the role of primary prevention cannot be discarded, the decrease in mortality has been attributed to improvements in pre-hospital and in hospital emergent care,[1] which we agree wholeheartedly with.

1.3 Stroke Risk Factors

Stroke risk factors surge from analytic epidemiology, and are an essential part of planning interventions to decrease incidence. These risk factors are usually separated into modifiable and non-modifiable, which helps to differentiate those that can be targets of preventive measures from those that cannot. A properly established risk factor requires multiple studies consistently supporting its association, compatible pathophysiological mechanisms, and ideally randomized controlled trials which show that intervention on these risk factors lowers stroke incidence.[1] Unfortunately, this is not always the case.

Known non-modifiable risk factors include age, male sex, African ancestry, family history of stroke, and genetic factors.[1] There are many modifiable risk factors, such as hypertension, diabetes, obesity, diet, and physical exercise.[1] A recent review of the burden of stroke and its risk factors in 188 countries by Feigin et al strongly suggests that modifiable risk factors account for 90% of total stroke burden, as measured by disability-adjusted life-years lost (DALYs).[13] The main contributors were behavioral risk factors such as smoking, lack of exercise and poor diet, followed by combined metabolic risk factors and pollution.[13] The INTER-STROKE study, a case-control study which followed 26 919 people from 32 countries between 2007 to 2015, also had similar results, showing that 10 modifiable risk factors accounted for 90% of stroke risk irrespective of age and sex.[26] These risk factors were Hypertension (OR 2.98), regular physical activity (0.60), apolipoprotein (Apo)B/ApoA1 ratio (OR 1.84), diet (OR 0.60), waist-to-hip ratio (OR 1.44), psychosocial factors (OR 2.20), smoking (OR 1.67), cardiac causes (OR 3.17), alcohol consumption (OR 2.09), and diabetes mellitus (OR 1.16).[26] We will discuss most major risk factors for stroke in this chapter.

1.3.1 Non-Modifiable Risk Factors

Age is the most important non-modifiable risk factor. It has been estimated that stroke risk doubles every decade after 55 years of age.[1] The increase with age has been consistently demonstrated across all studies to date.

Male sex is a risk factor for ischemic stroke in patients younger than 75 years of age, but not in those older.[4] This is probably due to the increased proportion on women in said age group, which leads to a higher number of cases.[1] For this reason, women also seem to have a higher total lifetime stroke risk.[27] Male sex has also been associated with intracerebral hematoma, whereas female sex is a risk factor for subarachnoid hemorrage.[1]

Those of African ancestry have an increased stroke risk. In the US, the Northern Manhattan Study (NOMAS) has shown an age adjusted incidence of stroke of 1.91/1000 people in blacks versus 0.88/1000 in whites.[28] In addition, in the US, both the NOMAS study and the BASIC project have shown an increased incidence in Mexican Americans.[28,29] Even though those of black race have an increased prevalence of some risk factors which could explain this association, such as hypertension, direct interpretation is difficult since separating race from socioeconomic status is not possible.[1]

A stroke before age 65 in either parent was associated with a threefold risk increase in offspring in the Framingham Heart Study.[29] This shows that there is a hereditary predisposition in some families. Recent studies suggest that the lower the age at the moment of stroke, female sex, large vessel disease and cardioembolic stroke for ischemic subtypes may have a stronger association.[4] The presence of a stroke on either parent increases the risk by a factor of approximately 2[1].

Some genetic mutations also confer a predisposition to stroke. For ischemic stroke, mutations in *HDAC, ABO, and TSPAN2* genes have been implicated in large vessel origin.[4] Other genes, such as *PTX2 and ZFHX3* have been related to cardioembolic ischemic stroke.[4] *FOXF2* mutations have been strongly related to small vessel disease.[4] Regarding hemorrhagic stroke, genes in the PMF1/BGLAP region have been linked to non-lobar ICH, and changes in Apolipoprotein E with lobar hematoma.[4] Even though these mutations, as well as others that are not currently known, increase stroke risk, familial risk cannot be attributed entirely to it. Other modifiable risk factors that can have an inherited component, such as hypertension or diabetes, as well as dietary habits in the family, certainly have interactions with the genetic component and affect the risk they confer.[1]

1.3.2 Modifiable Risk Factors

As mentioned before, modifiable causes may account for up to 90% of stroke risk[13,26].

1.3.3 Hypertension

The definition of hypertension has changed significantly in the past 20 years, and is still under discussion. Nonetheless, it is beyond discussion at this point that elevated values are a major modifiable risk factor for all stroke types.[4]

Moreover, several studies have shown that blood pressure control leads to reduced stroke risk, especially among patients with other comorbidities such as diabetes.[4] Some studies have also shown a larger benefit with intense blood pressure control, with target systolic pressure below 120 mmHg versus 140 mm Hg.[30] Nonetheless, there is still some disagreement on definitive target BP, and probably further randomized trials are necessary to achieve a definite consensus.

The effect of blood pressure is also variable between different populations. In African Americans, elevated blood pressure is responsible for approximately 20% of the increased stroke rate[31] whereas an increase in 10 mmHg lead to three times the increase in risk as in whites.[32]

1.3.4 Diabetes Mellitus

Diabetes is a significant risk factor across all ages and ethnicities. Furthermore, diabetic patients are likely to have other risk factors, leading to increased risk.[4] Diabetic women seem to have an increased risk compared to men. Prediabetes has also been associated with increased risk, but with a more modest effect.[4]

Diabetic patients are also at increased risk of recurrence.[33] Prognosis was significantly worse in diabetic women and younger patients.[4]

A definitive risk reduction has been shown in randomized control trials of treatment of people with prediabetes.[34] For diabetic patients, the treatment effects are difficult to separate from those of frequently associated comorbidities, such as hypertension. Nonetheless, there is no doubt that controlling both risk factors leads to decreased risk, and should thus be a therapeutic goal.[4]

1.3.5 Arrhythmias

Atrial fibrillation (AF) has long been established as a risk factor for cardioembolic stroke, with a fivefold increase in risk and increased attributed burden with age.[4] AF is discovered in up to 23% of cryptogenic stroke patients with a 3 to 4 week follow up, since AF is often asymptomatic.[4]

Several factors increase the risk of stroke in patients with AF. These include age, hypertension, DM, previous stroke or TIA, vascular disease, and female sex.[35,36]

1.3.6 Lipids

There is no clear association between different lipid subtypes at this point. In the future, randomized trials will be necessary to determine the association of cholesterol, triglycerides, and other sub fractions with specific stroke subtypes, and the treatment effect for targeted drugs.[37,38,39,40,41]

1.3.7 Smoking

Smoking is, together with high blood pressure, the strongest modifiable factor both in primary and secondary stroke prevention. Strong countrywide tobacco control policies being instituted in the previous years in several different countries will hopefully lead to a decrease in stroke in the future.

Smokers have a two- to fourfold increase in stroke risk, compared to nonsmokers. Quitting after 10 years has been shown to reduce this risk significantly.[42,43] Heavy smoking has also been associated with increased risk.[43,44] Furthermore, a marked decrease in risk has been shown several years after quitting, with light smokers having the same risk as nonsmokers after a period of 5 years in some studies.[4]

Smoking might also synergize with other risk factors, such as hypertension.[45] This is likely related to both the direct effect of smoking on the body and the lifestyle of heavy smokers.

Second hand smoke has also been shown to be a dose-dependent risk factor for stroke, albeit the risk seems to be lower than active smoking.[46,47,48]

1.3.8 Exercise

Several studies have shown a clear benefit related to regular physical activity. The estimated reduction in stroke risk is up to 50% in some studies.[49,50,51] The benefit seems to be dose- dependent, with at least moderate to vigorous activity required for a clear benefit, although modest exercise might also be beneficial.[50,52,53,54] Most of the benefits attributed to exercise can probably be explained by the positive effect it has on other risk factors, such as hypertension and obesity.

1.3.9 Nutrition

One study has shown a clear benefit related to adhering to a calorie-unrestricted Mediterranean-style diet, with increased content of nuts and olive oil, fruits and cereals, and a reduced consumption of dairy products, meats and sweets.[55] Although this was a randomized trial, participants were middle-aged or elderly Spanish people with at least 3 risk factors for cardiovascular disease or diabetes, and there are several limitations that have been recognized by the authors.[55] Thus, strictly speaking, this intervention was effective in this population, and the benefits for adoption of this diet in younger patients, those without risk factors, or those with other comorbidities is unclear. It is very likely that a Mediterranean style diet in those populations will have a benefit, albeit small. Further studies are required to prove this.

Another recent study from a Danish cohort has shown some benefit to adhering to a Nordic diet, with increased consumption of fish, fruits, root vegetables and oatmeal.[56] Thus, both diets may be viable options for prevention of stroke. More important than these diets might be what they have in common, with reduced consumption of red meats, bread and flour derivatives, and sweets; these items could be possible targets of health policy. Future studies might be necessary to address whether the relevant elements of these dietary modifications are the elements whose consumption is increased, or those avoided.

Finally, specific dietary supplements might be relevant for stroke prevention in some populations. For example, in a study involving Chinese adults with hypertension, the addition of a folate supplement decreased stroke risk.[57] Although the effect of folates may not be significant in countries where food is enriched with it, it may be a reasonable intervention in those countries not adhering to this norm.

1.3.10 Chronic Kidney Disease

It has been consistently shown that low glomerular filtration rate is associated with increased stroke incidence, severity, morbidity and mortality. Moreover, this effect seems to increase the worse the filtration rate is.[58,59,60,61]

1.3.11 Oral Estrogen Therapy

Data from randomized clinical trials suggest that estrogen replacement therapy, whether alone or associated with progestin, increases stroke risk in postmenopausal women.[62,63,64,65]

When used as an oral contraceptive, estrogen increases stroke risk in women. This increase seems dose-dependent.[66,67,68,69] The association of migraine with auras or smoking also increases this risk significantly. The presence of all three factors confers nine times the risk, and should be avoided whenever possible.[70,71]

1.3.12 Sleep Apnea

In recent years, this frequent pathology in middle-aged people[72,73] has been associated with increased stroke risk, and represents a potential intervention to minimize stroke while improving quality of life. Studies suggest that the increase in risk depends on the severity of the apnea and affects males more than females.[74,75,76] It has also been linked with an increase in morbidity after stroke[77] and mortality.[78,79,80]

In addition, obstructive sleep apnea has an extremely high prevalence in stroke survivors, of over 50%.[74,81,82] This is a very significant finding, since treatment might be a relevant factor in secondary stroke prevention for these patients.

At this point, further research is needed to determine whether current sleep apnea therapy is effective as primary or secondary stroke prevention with strong evidence levels.

1.3.13 Perinatal and Childhood Strokes

Even though its usually regarded as an infrequent occurrence, cerebrovascular disease is among the top 10 causes of death in the pediatric population.[83] Mortality is highest in the first year of life, with 7.8 deaths/100000, with an increased risk in males and those of African ancestry.[83]

Pediatric strokes are classified as perinatal when they occur between 28 weeks of gestation and 28 days of life, and as childhood strokes if they occur on older children.[83] The incidence of neonatal stroke is roughly 1 in 4000 live births per year,[83] and is a significant cause of morbidity and mortality.

The incidence of childhood stroke, increases with age, from 2–3 cases/100000 person-year for those under 5 years of age to 8 cases/100000 person-year for those under 14 years of age.[84] The relationship between ischemic and hemorrhagic stroke during childhood is approximately 1:1, unlike in adults.[85,86,87]

Known independent risk factors for perinatal stroke include infertility, preeclampsia, prolonged rupture of membranes, and chorioamnionitis,[4] and common associations are acute systemic disease (infectious and noninfectious), and prothrombotic states.[84]

In older children, the most common risk factor is arteriopathy, found in 50% of all cases, followed by congenital or acquired cardiopathy (24%), and prothrombotic states and hematologic diseases (20%-50%).[88,89] Congenital cardiopathy increases stroke risk by 19-fold.[90] Migraine also seems to be a risk factor for stroke in teenagers. In one US study, adolescents with migraines had a three times higher risk of stroke, but not younger children.[91] A 2005 metanalysis in adults and young adults has shown that it may be a significant independent risk factor for stroke, with approximately a two-fold increase in risk, which goes up to 8 fold in the presence of oral contraceptives.[92] Even

though this study did not investigate a pediatric population, it raises powerful concerns, given that adolescents are starting earlier with hormonal contraceptives, which could lead to an increase in pediatric stroke if appropriate measures are not taken.

Trauma to the head or neck is also a risk factor for ischemic stroke, present in 10% of pediatric ischemic stroke patients.[93] Even though this is the reported percentage, in daily practice in our center traumatic arterial dissections in pediatric patients seem to be much higher. A possible explanation may be the underestimation of this pathology due to sub-utilization of endovascular diagnostic techniques.

In addition, recent infection (in the previous days) seems to increase stroke risk.[93,94] Finally, herpesvirus infection has been strongly linked to ischemic stroke in a study with 326 patients.[95] It must be noted that most infections were sub-clinical in this study.

Recurrence rates in pediatric stroke have been estimated at 10% at 5 years, and may be even as high as 25%.[96,97] Secondary prevention and strict follow-up is mandatory to prevent and control this.

1.4 Conclusion

Overall, rather than looking at each risk factor as a single element to correct, we believe that effective stroke prevention requires a lifestyle change, which is a long-term investment. This change requires both encouragement at the personal level by primary care physicians as well as public health policies that make it easier for people to exercise, reduce smoking and eat healthier diets. Moreover, improving outcomes requires better and faster access to healthcare, appropriate treatment, rehabilitation and secondary prevention. We are convinced this should be a worldwide effort of the medical community, since this is a true pandemic running unchecked.

References

[1] Bousser M-G, Mas J-L. Accidents Vasculaires Cérébraux. DOIN; 2009

[2] Feigin VL, Krishnamurthi RV, Parmar P, et al. GBD 2013 Writing Group, GBD 2013 Stroke Panel Experts Group. Update on the Global Burden of Ischemic and Hemorrhagic Stroke in 1990–2013: The GBD 2013 Study. Neuroepidemiology. 2015; 45(3):161–176

[3] Feigin VL, Forouzanfar MH, Krishnamurthi R, et al. Global Burden of Diseases, Injuries, and Risk Factors Study 2010

(GBD 2010) and the GBD Stroke Experts Group. Global and regional burden of stroke during 1990–2010: findings from the Global Burden of Disease Study 2010. Lancet. 2014; 383 (9913):245–254

[4] Benjamin EJ, Blaha MJ, Chiuve SE, et al. American Heart Association Statistics Committee and Stroke Statistics Subcommittee. Heart Disease and Stroke Statistics-2017 Update: A Report From the American Heart Association. Circulation. 2017; 135(10):e146–e603

[5] Centers for Disease Control and Prevention (CDC). Prevalence of stroke–United States, 2006–2010. MMWR Morb Mortal Wkly Rep. 2012; 61(20):379–382

[6] Howard VJ, McClure LA, Meschia JF, Pulley L, Orr SC, Friday GH. High prevalence of stroke symptoms among persons without a diagnosis of stroke or transient ischemic attack in a general population: the REasons for Geographic And Racial Differences in Stroke (REGARDS) study. Arch Intern Med. 2006; 166(18):1952–1958

[7] Ovbiagele B, Goldstein LB, Higashida RT, et al. American Heart Association Advocacy Coordinating Committee and Stroke Council. Forecasting the future of stroke in the United States: a policy statement from the American Heart Association and American Stroke Association. Stroke. 2013; 44(8):2361–2375

[8] Reeves MJ, Bushnell CD, Howard G, et al. Sex differences in stroke: epidemiology, clinical presentation, medical care, and outcomes. Lancet Neurol. 2008; 7(10):915–926

[9] Krishnamurthi RV, Feigin VL, Forouzanfar MH, et al. Global Burden of Diseases, Injuries, Risk Factors Study 2010 (GBD 2010), GBD Stroke Experts Group. Global and regional burden of first-ever ischaemic and haemorrhagic stroke during 1990–2010: findings from the Global Burden of Disease Study 2010. Lancet Glob Health. 2013; 1(5):e259–e281

[10] Béjot Y, Daubail B, Giroud M. Epidemiology of stroke and transient ischemic attacks: Current knowledge and perspectives. Rev Neurol (Paris). 2016; 172(1):59–68

[11] Kleindorfer DO, Khoury J, Moomaw CJ, et al. Stroke incidence is decreasing in whites but not in blacks: a population-based estimate of temporal trends in stroke incidence from the Greater Cincinnati/Northern Kentucky Stroke Study. Stroke. 2010; 41(7):1326–1331

[12] Thrift AG, Cadilhac DA, Thayabaranathan T, et al. Global stroke statistics. Int J Stroke. 2014; 9(1):6–18

[13] Feigin VL, Roth GA, Naghavi M, et al. Global Burden of Diseases, Injuries and Risk Factors Study 2013 and Stroke Experts Writing Group. Global burden of stroke and risk factors in 188 countries, during 1990–2013: a systematic analysis for the Global Burden of Disease Study 2013. Lancet Neurol. 2016; 15(9):913–924

[14] Hankey GJ. Impact of Treatment of People with Transient Ischaemic Attacks on Stroke Incidence and Public Health. Cerebrovasc Dis. 1996; 6(1):26–33

[15] Johnston SC, Fayad PB, Gorelick PB, et al. Prevalence and knowledge of transient ischemic attack among US adults. Neurology. 2003; 60(9):1429–1434

[16] Johnston SC, Gress DR, Browner WS, Sidney S. Short-term prognosis after emergency department diagnosis of TIA. JAMA. 2000; 284(22):2901–2906

[17] Wu CM, McLaughlin K, Lorenzetti DL, Hill MD, Manns BJ, Ghali WA. Early risk of stroke after transient ischemic attack: a systematic review and meta-analysis. Arch Intern Med. 2007; 167(22):2417–2422

[18] Giles MF, Rothwell PM. Risk of stroke early after transient ischaemic attack: a systematic review and meta-analysis. Lancet Neurol. 2007; 6(12):1063–1072

[19] Luengo-Fernandez R, Paul NLM, Gray AM, et al. Oxford Vascular Study. Population-based study of disability and institutionalization after transient ischemic attack and stroke: 10-year results of the Oxford Vascular Study. Stroke. 2013; 44 (10):2854–2861

[20] Pennlert J, Eriksson M, Carlberg B, Wiklund PG. Long-term risk and predictors of recurrent stroke beyond the acute phase. Stroke. 2014; 45(6):1839–1841

[21] Feng W, Hendry RM, Adams RJ. Risk of recurrent stroke, myocardial infarction, or death in hospitalized stroke patients. Neurology. 2010; 74(7):588–593

[22] Hong K-S, Yegiaian S, Lee M, Lee J, Saver JL. Declining stroke and vascular event recurrence rates in secondary prevention trials over the past 50 years and consequences for current trial design. Circulation. 2011; 123(19):2111–2119

[23] Allen NB, Holford TR, Bracken MB, et al. Trends in one-year recurrent ischemic stroke among the elderly in the USA: 1994–2002. Cerebrovasc Dis. 2010; 30(5):525–532

[24] Pezzini A, Grassi M, Lodigiani C, et al. Italian Project on Stroke in Young Adults (IPSYS) Investigators. Predictors of long-term recurrent vascular events after ischemic stroke at young age: the Italian Project on Stroke in Young Adults. Circulation. 2014; 129(16):1668–1676

[25] Koton S, Schneider ALC, Rosamond WD, et al. Stroke incidence and mortality trends in US communities, 1987 to 2011. JAMA. 2014; 312(3):259–268

[26] O'Donnell MJ, Chin SL, Rangarajan S, et al. INTERSTROKE investigators. Global and regional effects of potentially modifiable risk factors associated with acute stroke in 32 countries (INTERSTROKE): a case-control study. Lancet. 2016; 388 (10046):761–775

[27] Wolf PA, D'Agostino RB, O'Neal MA, et al. Secular trends in stroke incidence and mortality. The Framingham Study. Stroke. 1992; 23(11):1551–1555

[28] White H, Boden-Albala B, Wang C, et al. Ischemic stroke subtype incidence among whites, blacks, and Hispanics: the Northern Manhattan Study. Circulation. 2005; 111(10): 1327–1331

[29] Morgenstern LB, Smith MA, Lisabeth LD, et al. Excess stroke in Mexican Americans compared with non-Hispanic Whites: the Brain Attack Surveillance in Corpus Christi Project. Am J Epidemiol. 2004; 160(4):376–383

[30] Perkovic V, Rodgers A. Redefining Blood-Pressure Targets–SPRINT Starts the Marathon. N Engl J Med. 2015; 373(22): 2175–2178

[31] Howard G, Cushman M, Kissela BM, et al. REasons for Geographic And Racial Differences in Stroke (REGARDS) Investigators. Traditional risk factors as the underlying cause of racial disparities in stroke: lessons from the half-full (empty?) glass. Stroke. 2011; 42(12):3369–3375

[32] Howard G, Lackland DT, Kleindorfer DO, et al. Racial differences in the impact of elevated systolic blood pressure on stroke risk. JAMA Intern Med. 2013; 173(1):46–51

[33] Shou J, Zhou L, Zhu S, Zhang X. Diabetes is an Independent Risk Factor for Stroke Recurrence in Stroke Patients: A Meta-analysis. J Stroke Cerebrovasc Dis. 2015; 24(9):1961–1968

[34] Hopper I, Billah B, Skiba M, Krum H. Prevention of diabetes and reduction in major cardiovascular events in studies of subjects with prediabetes: meta-analysis of randomised controlled clinical trials. Eur J Cardiovasc Prev Rehabil. 2011; 18 (6):813–823

[35] Gage BF, Waterman AD, Shannon W, Boechler M, Rich MW, Radford MJ. Validation of clinical classification schemes for predicting stroke: results from the National Registry of Atrial Fibrillation. JAMA. 2001; 285(22):2864–2870

[36] Lip GYH, Nieuwlaat R, Pisters R, Lane DA, Crijns HJGM. Refining clinical risk stratification for predicting stroke and thromboembolism in atrial fibrillation using a novel risk factor-based approach: the euro heart survey on atrial fibrillation. Chest. 2010; 137(2):263–272

[37] Amarenco P, Labreuche J, Touboul P-J. High-density lipoprotein-cholesterol and risk of stroke and carotid atherosclerosis: a systematic review. Atherosclerosis. 2008; 196(2):489–496

[38] Zhang Y, Tuomilehto J, Jousilahti P, Wang Y, Antikainen R, Hu G. Total and High-Density Lipoprotein Cholesterol and Stroke Risk. http://stroke.ahajournals.org/content/strokeaha/early/2012/04/10/STROKEAHA.111.646778.full.pdf. Accessed December 28, 2017

[39] Horenstein RB, Smith DE, Mosca L. Cholesterol predicts stroke mortality in the Women's Pooling Project. Stroke. 2002; 33(7):1863–1868

[40] Lewington S, Whitlock G, Clarke R, et al. Prospective Studies Collaboration. Blood cholesterol and vascular mortality by age, sex, and blood pressure: a meta-analysis of individual data from 61 prospective studies with 55,000 vascular deaths. Lancet. 2007; 370(9602):1829–1839

[41] Wang X, Dong Y, Qi X, Huang C, Hou L. Cholesterol levels and risk of hemorrhagic stroke: a systematic review and meta-analysis. Stroke. 2013; 44(7):1833–1839

[42] Shah RS, Cole JW. Smoking and stroke: the more you smoke the more you stroke. Expert Rev Cardiovasc Ther. 2010; 8(7):917–932

[43] Goldstein LB, Bushnell CD, Adams RJ, et al. American Heart Association Stroke Council, Council on Cardiovascular Nursing, Council on Epidemiology and Prevention, Council for High Blood Pressure Research, Council on Peripheral Vascular Disease, and Interdisciplinary Council on Quality of Care and Outcomes Research. Guidelines for the primary prevention of stroke: a guideline for healthcare professionals from the American Heart Association/American Stroke Association. Stroke. 2011; 42(2):517–584

[44] Bhat VM, Cole JW, Sorkin JD, et al. Dose-response relationship between cigarette smoking and risk of ischemic stroke in young women. Stroke. 2008; 39(9):2439–2443

[45] Nakamura K, Barzi F, Lam T-H, et al. Asia Pacific Cohort Studies Collaboration. Cigarette smoking, systolic blood pressure, and cardiovascular diseases in the Asia-Pacific region. Stroke. 2008; 39(6):1694–1702

[46] Malek AM, Cushman M, Lackland DT, Howard G, McClure LA, McClure LA. Secondhand Smoke Exposure and Stroke: The Reasons for Geographic and Racial Differences in Stroke (REGARDS) Study. Am J Prev Med. 2015; 49(6):e89–e97

[47] Oono IP, Mackay DF, Pell JP. Meta-analysis of the association between secondhand smoke exposure and stroke. J Public Health (Oxf). 2011; 33(4):496–502

[48] Lee PN, Forey BA. Environmental tobacco smoke exposure and risk of stroke in nonsmokers: a review with meta-analysis. J Stroke Cerebrovasc Dis. 2006; 15(5):190–201

[49] McDonnell MN, Hillier SL, Hooker SP, Le A, Judd SE, Howard VJ. Physical activity frequency and risk of incident stroke in a national US study of blacks and whites. Stroke. 2013; 44(9):2519–2524

[50] Bell EJ, Lutsey PL, Windham BG, Folsom AR. Physical activity and cardiovascular disease in African Americans in Atherosclerosis Risk in Communities. Med Sci Sports Exerc. 2013; 45(5):901–907

[51] Tikk K, Sookthai D, Monni S, et al. Primary preventive potential for stroke by avoidance of major lifestyle risk factors: the European Prospective Investigation into Cancer and Nutrition-Heidelberg cohort. Stroke. 2014; 45(7):2041–2046

[52] Willey JZ, Moon YP, Paik MC, Boden-Albala B, Sacco RL, Elkind MSV. Physical activity and risk of ischemic stroke in the Northern Manhattan Study. Neurology. 2009; 73(21):1774–1779

[53] Hooker SP, Sui X, Colabianchi N, et al. Cardiorespiratory fitness as a predictor of fatal and nonfatal stroke in asymptomatic women and men. Stroke. 2008; 39(11):2950–2957

[54] Hu G, Sarti C, Jousilahti P, Silventoinen K, Barengo NC, Tuomilehto J. Leisure time, occupational, and commuting physical activity and the risk of stroke. Stroke. 2005; 36(9):1994–1999

[55] Estruch R, Ros E, Salas-Salvadó J, et al. PREDIMED Study Investigators. Primary prevention of cardiovascular disease with a Mediterranean diet. N Engl J Med. 2013; 368(14):1279–1290

[56] Hansen CP, Overvad K, Kyrø C, et al. Adherence to a Healthy Nordic Diet and Risk of Stroke: A Danish Cohort Study. Stroke. 2017; 48(2):259–264

[57] Huo Y, Li J, Qin X, et al. CSPPT Investigators. Efficacy of folic acid therapy in primary prevention of stroke among adults with hypertension in China: the CSPPT randomized clinical trial. JAMA. 2015; 313(13):1325–1335

[58] Lee M, Saver JL, Chang K-H, Liao H-W, Chang S-C, Ovbiagele B. Low glomerular filtration rate and risk of stroke: meta-analysis. BMJ. 2010; 341:c4249

[59] Holzmann MJ, Aastveit A, Hammar N, Jungner I, Walldius G, Holme I. Renal dysfunction increases the risk of ischemic and hemorrhagic stroke in the general population. Ann Med. 2012; 44(6):607–615

[60] Molshatzki N, Orion D, Tsabari R, et al. Chronic kidney disease in patients with acute intracerebral hemorrhage: association with large hematoma volume and poor outcome. Cerebrovasc Dis. 2011; 31(3):271–277

[61] Mahmoodi BK, Yatsuya H, Matsushita K, et al. Association of kidney disease measures with ischemic versus hemorrhagic strokes: pooled analyses of 4 prospective community-based cohorts. Stroke. 2014; 45(7):1925–1931

[62] Rossouw JE, Anderson GL, Prentice RL, et al. Writing Group for the Women's Health Initiative Investigators. Risks and benefits of estrogen plus progestin in healthy postmenopausal women: principal results From the Women's Health Initiative randomized controlled trial. JAMA. 2002; 288(3):321–333

[63] Hendrix SL, Wassertheil-Smoller S, Johnson KC, et al. WHI Investigators. Effects of conjugated equine estrogen on stroke in the Women's Health Initiative. Circulation. 2006; 113(20):2425–2434

[64] Wassertheil-Smoller S, Hendrix SL, Limacher M, et al. WHI Investigators. Effect of estrogen plus progestin on stroke in postmenopausal women: the Women's Health Initiative: a randomized trial. JAMA. 2003; 289(20):2673–2684

[65] Heart T, Hers ERS, Simon JA, et al. Clinical Investigation and Reports Postmenopausal Hormone Therapy and Risk of Stroke. Circulation. 2001; •••:638–643

[66] Renoux C, Dell'aniello S, Garbe E, Suissa S. Transdermal and oral hormone replacement therapy and the risk of stroke: a nested case-control study. BMJ. 2010; 340:c2519

[67] Gillum LA, Mamidipudi SK, Johnston SC. Ischemic stroke risk with oral contraceptives: A meta-analysis. JAMA. 2000; 284(1):72–78

[68] Gillum LA, Johnston SC. Oral contraceptives and stroke risk: the debate continues. Lancet Neurol. 2004; 3(8):453–454

[69] Roach REJ, Helmerhorst FM, Lijfering WM, Algra A, Dekkers OM. Combined oral contraceptives: the risk of myocardial infarction and ischemic stroke. In: Roach REJ, ed. Cochrane

Database of Systematic Reviews. Chichester, UK: John Wiley & Sons, Ltd; 2014. doi:10.1002/14651858.CD011054

[70] MacClellan LR, Giles W, Cole J, et al. Probable migraine with visual aura and risk of ischemic stroke: the stroke prevention in young women study. Stroke. 2007; 38(9):2438–2445

[71] Schürks M, Rist PM, Bigal ME, Buring JE, Lipton RB, Kurth T. Migraine and cardiovascular disease: systematic review and meta-analysis. BMJ. 2009; 339:b3914

[72] Peppard PE, Young T, Barnet JH, Palta M, Hagen EW, Hla KM. Increased prevalence of sleep-disordered breathing in adults. Am J Epidemiol. 2013; 177(9):1006–1014

[73] Chen X, Wang R, Zee P, et al. Racial/Ethnic Differences in Sleep Disturbances: The Multi-Ethnic Study of Atherosclerosis (MESA). Sleep (Basel). 2015; 38(6):877–888

[74] Johnson KG, Johnson DC. Frequency of sleep apnea in stroke and TIA patients: a meta-analysis. J Clin Sleep Med. 2010; 6 (2):131–137

[75] Loke YK, Brown JWL, Kwok CS, Niruban A, Myint PK. Association of obstructive sleep apnea with risk of serious cardiovascular events: a systematic review and meta-analysis. Circ Cardiovasc Qual Outcomes. 2012; 5(5):720–728

[76] Li M, Hou W-S, Zhang X-W, Tang Z-Y. Obstructive sleep apnea and risk of stroke: a meta-analysis of prospective studies. Int J Cardiol. 2014; 172(2):466–469

[77] Turkington PM, Bamford J, Wanklyn P, Elliott MW, Elliott MW. Prevalence and predictors of upper airway obstruction in the first 24 hours after acute stroke. Stroke. 2002; 33(8): 2037–2042

[78] Martínez-García MÁ, Soler-Cataluña JJ, Ejarque-Martínez L, et al. Continuous positive airway pressure treatment reduces mortality in patients with ischemic stroke and obstructive sleep apnea: a 5-year follow-up study. Am J Respir Crit Care Med. 2009; 180(1):36–41

[79] Parra O, Arboix A, Montserrat JM, Quintó L, Bechich S, García-Eroles L. Sleep-related breathing disorders: impact on mortality of cerebrovascular disease. Eur Respir J. 2004; 24(2): 267–272

[80] Sahlin C, Sandberg O, Gustafson Y, et al. Obstructive sleep apnea is a risk factor for death in patients with stroke: a 10-year follow-up. Arch Intern Med. 2008; 168(3):297–301

[81] Johnson DA, Lisabeth L, Lewis TT, et al. The Contribution of Psychosocial Stressors to Sleep among African Americans in the Jackson Heart Study. Sleep (Basel). 2016; 39(7):1411–1419

[82] Broadley SA, Jørgensen L, Cheek A, et al. Early investigation and treatment of obstructive sleep apnoea after acute stroke. J Clin Neurosci. 2007; 14(4):328–333

[83] Lynch JK, Hirtz DG, Deveber G, Nelson KB. Report of the National Institute of Neurological Disorders and Stroke Workshop on Perinatal and Childhood Stroke. Pediatr Blvd. 2002;109116

[84] González G, Russi ME, Crosa R. Accidente cerebrovascular en la infancia y adolescencia. In: González G, Arroyo H, Crosa R, Russi ME, eds. Accidente Cerebrovascular En La Infancia Y Adolescencia. 1a Edicion. Buenos Aires: Ediciones Journal; 2011:1–14

[85] Kleindorfer D, Khoury J, Kissela B, et al. Temporal trends in the incidence and case fatality of stroke in children and adolescents. J Child Neurol. 2006; 21(5):415–418

[86] Agrawal N, Johnston SC, Wu YW, Sidney S, Fullerton HJ. Imaging data reveal a higher pediatric stroke incidence than prior US estimates. Stroke. 2009; 40(11):3415–3421

[87] Broderick J, Brott T, Kothari R, et al. The Greater Cincinnati/ Northern Kentucky Stroke Study: preliminary first-ever and total incidence rates of stroke among blacks. Stroke. 1998; 29 (2):415–421

[88] Mackay MT, Wiznitzer M, Benedict SL, Lee KJ, Deveber GA, Ganesan V, International Pediatric Stroke Study Group. Arterial ischemic stroke risk factors: the International Pediatric Stroke Study. Ann Neurol. 2011; 69(1):130–140

[89] Ganesan V, Prengler M, McShane MA, Wade AM, Kirkham FJ. Investigation of risk factors in children with arterial ischemic stroke. Ann Neurol. 2003; 53(2):167–173

[90] Fox CK, Sidney S, Fullerton HJ. Community-based case-control study of childhood stroke risk associated with congenital heart disease. Stroke. 2015; 46(2):336–340

[91] Gelfand AA, Fullerton HJ, Jacobson A, et al. Is migraine a risk factor for pediatric stroke? Cephalalgia. 2015; 35(14): 1252–1260

[92] Etminan M, Takkouche B, Isorna FC, Samii A. Risk of ischaemic stroke in people with migraine: systematic review and meta-analysis of observational studies. BMJ. 2005; 330 (7482):63

[93] Hills NK, Johnston SC, Sidney S, Zielinski BA, Fullerton HJ. Recent trauma and acute infection as risk factors for childhood arterial ischemic stroke. Ann Neurol. 2012; 72(6):850–858

[94] Fonarow GC, Smith EE, Saver JL, et al. Timeliness of tissue-type plasminogen activator therapy in acute ischemic stroke: patient characteristics, hospital factors, and outcomes associated with door-to-needle times within 60 minutes. Circulation. 2011; 123(7):750–758

[95] Elkind MSV, Hills NK, Glaser CA, et al. VIPS Investigators*. Herpesvirus Infections and Childhood Arterial Ischemic Stroke: Results of the VIPS Study. Circulation. 2016; 133(8): 732–741

[96] Danchaivijitr N, Cox TC, Saunders DE, Ganesan V. Evolution of cerebral arteriopathies in childhood arterial ischemic stroke. Ann Neurol. 2006; 59(4):620–626

[97] Tuppin P, Samson S, Woimant F, Chabrier S. Management and 2-year follow-up of children aged 29 days to 17 years hospitalized for a first stroke in France (2009–2010). Arch Pediatr. 2014; 21(12):1305–1315

2 Intravenous Thrombolysis in Stroke. The Organization of Stroke Centers

Sheila Cristina Ouriques Martins, Ana Claudia de Souza, Leonardo Augusto Carbonera, and Carlos Batista

Abstract

The burden of stroke is a challenge to the health-care systems worldwide, for its elevated incidence and morbimortality. Given the rise of reperfusion therapies specially intravenous rtPA , the patients needed to arrive in a tertiary center within the therapeutic window, in order to receive adequate treatment. Therefore, stroke systems of care started to be developed, and the increasing volume of stroke patients demanded structuration and organization of the tertiary hospitals for achieving better outcomes. An expressive number of countries and regions with their singular political, cultural and socioeconomical background engaged in this task. This chapter brings an overview of the optimal pathway for acute stroke care with the use of IV-tPA and briefly describes the process of implementation of Stroke Units in some developing and developed countries.

Keywords: stroke centers, stroke units, stroke systems of care, developing countries, developed countries, tissue plasminogen activator

Stroke is the second cause of mortality and the major cause of disability in the world [1]. Despite the great advances on prevention, diagnosis and treatment in the last decades, there is still a gap between scientific evidences and their implementation, mainly in low and middle income countries. The proof of the benefit of intravenous (IV) thrombolysis for ischemic stroke in the NINDS trial [2] and its approval by the Food and Drug Administration (FDA) in 1996 promoted the development of the stroke treatment system around the world, along with stroke centers (SCs) organization and implementation of acute phase strategies, followed by organization of pre-hospital Emergency Medical Services (EMS), education campaigns for the community and health care professionals and development of a rehabilitation network.

The organization of the stroke care system is a factor that directly influences patient outcome and reduces both mortality and disability. There is an immense variety of stroke care models around the world. To diminish the disparity of care between the countries, the World Stroke Organization (WSO) is highly committed to detecting barriers that prevent adequate care and suggesting the implementation of evidence-based interventions in stroke care.[3]

Strategies that modify the natural history of stroke include treatment with IV thrombolysis and organization of SCs to develop into Stroke Units (SUs). The scope of this chapter is to discuss these two strategies.

2.1 Intravenous Thrombolysis

Ischemic stroke, which accounts for 85% of the stroke cases, occurs when there is an interruption of blood flow in the brain. Prompt reperfusion of the occluded vessel can limit the ischemic area and can reduce or even avoid the disability. Therefore, the most important aspect of stroke management is fast diagnosis and treatment in a safe, monitored place with well-trained staff. The recombinant tissue plasminogen activator (rtPA) is the only approved systemic treatment for acute stroke until 4, 5 hours of symptom onset.[4] Other drugs are being tested (i.e. tenecteplase), but we still lack sufficient data to justify their use.

2.1.1 Acute Management

The current stroke management depends on recognition of the disease as a medical urgency. A stroke referral hospital must be aware of the necessity to prioritize the care of these patients, which leads to rapid diagnostic investigation and specific treatment.

Detection, Diagnosis and Differential Diagnosis

Every patient presenting with neurological focal deficit of sudden onset must be evaluated as a possible case of stroke. The most frequent conditions that mimic an ischemic stroke are conversion disorders, undetected seizures, confusional state, meningitis/encephalitis, hypertensive encephalopathy, syncope, toxic/metabolic disturbances (e.g., hypoglycemia) complicated migraine, brain tumors and subdural hematoma. These conditions can be ruled out in the emergency evaluation.

Those conditions, which are also known as Stroke Mimics, were identified in approximately 3% of the cases in two series of patients that received rtPA. Most of those patients had conversion disorders.[5,6] However, there was no evidence of complication secondary to the thrombolysis. Recently, in a register of 512 patients treated with rtPA until 3 hours of symptom onset, 21% were classified at the end of the workup as suffering from stroke mimics.[7] In this cohort, the majority of the patients had seizures, complicated migraines and conversion disorders, and none of them had symptomatic intracranial hemorrhage. Although the IV thrombolysis apparently does no harm to patients without a stroke, it is recommended to have a rate of less than 3% of stroke mimics receiving rtPA, when using only a CT scan to select the patient.[8] The means to find the balance between fast treatment and accurate diagnosis continue to evolve.

Acute Phase Evaluation

It is fundamental to establish the exact time of symptom onset when a stroke is suspected. By convention, it is the last moment in which the patient was seen without deficits; consequently, if the patient wakes up in the morning with stroke signs, the last time the patient was seen asymptomatic would be before bedtime.

After detecting a potential stroke patient on admission at the ED and defining the time of symptom onset, a medical and nursing evaluation should be promptly demanded. While the emergency physician confirms the stroke hypothesis and calls the neurologist for an evaluation, the nurse places two peripheral venous lines, monitors vital signs and checks capillary glycemia. After that, the physician orders a CT scan, an electrocardiogram and laboratory tests. In some hospitals, to expedite the process, as soon as the pre-hospital EMS already recognizes the possibility of a stroke, the patient is moved right away to Radiology. There the medical assessment is completed and, if positive for stroke, a bolus of rtPA is administered.

The neurological evaluation must be rapid and comprehensive. The use of assessment scales allows the evaluation of a great number of components of the neurological examination in a short period of time. The most frequently used scale for the quantification of neurological deficit is the National Institute of Health Stroke Scale (NIHSS) (▶ Table 2.1), ranging from zero (no deficit) to 42 (complete deficit). It can be performed by neurolo-

gist, emergency physician, nurse or any other healthcare professional. The use of a standardized scale facilitates the communication between professionals, contributes to estimating prognosis and helps to decide reperfusion strategies.

Ancillary Testing in the Acute Phase

All stroke patients must have an electrocardiogram, blood and platelet count, prothrombin time (PT) with international normalized ratio (INR) and activated partial thromboplastin time (aPTT), serum electrolyte dosage (sodium, potassium), serum urea and creatinine, and glycemia. Since 2007, it is no longer necessary to wait for laboratory results to initiate thrombolysis. Before that date, checking the platelet count was recommended before rtPA infusion, delaying the start of the treatment. The probability of a platelet count below $100.000/mm^3$ in a patient with acute stroke is 0,3% if neither history nor clinical features are suggestive of blood diathesis. PT and aTTP must be checked before thrombolysis only in patients on anticoagulants (warfarin and unfractionated heparin, respectively). If there is no history of use of those medications, thrombolysis must be initiated, and the laboratory results will be checked during the rtPA infusion.[9,10]

In patients on dabigatran, either normal thrombin time (TT), ecarin clotting time (ET) or aPTT can be performed to rule out significant activity. Considering TT and ET are not widely available in the emergency setting, a history of missing the last dose of dabigatran plus a normal aPTT may permit to proceed with thrombolysis, weighing risks versus benefits for each single case. There are no reliable tests to verify the activity of rivaroxaban and apixaban, so patients on those medications are excluded from the thrombolytic therapy – unless the patient has not been taking the medication for the last 48 hours.[9]

Imaging in the Acute Phase

The non-contrast CT (NCCT) brain scan is indispensable in the emergency evaluation of patients with acute stroke. It identifies 90–95% of subarachnoid hemorrhages and almost 100% of intraparenchymal hemorrhages and helps to rule out non-vascular causes for the neurological symptoms.

Early signs of infarction or arterial occlusion on NCCT can be observed in the first hours after a stroke (60% of cases within 2 hours from symptom onset[11]). Hyperdense artery sign in the area

Table 2.1 National Institute of Health Stroke Scale (NIHSS)

Description	Score
1a. Level of Consciousness	0 = Alert; keenly responsive. 1 = Not alert; but arousable by minor stimulation to obey, answer, or respond. 2 = Not alert; requires repeated stimulation to attend, or is obtunded and requires strong or painful stimulation to make movements (not stereotyped) 3 = Responds only with reflex motor or autonomic effects or totally unresponsive, flaccid and areflexic.
1b. LOC Questions	0 = Answers both questions correctly. 1 = Answers one question correctly. 2 = Answers neither question correctly.
1c. LOC Commands	0 = Performs both tasks correctly. 1 = Performs one task correctly. 2 = Performs neither task correctly.
2. Best Gaze	0 = Normal. Able to move both eyes left to right across midline. 1 = Partial gaze palsy. Gaze is abnormal in one or both eyes, but neither forced deviation nor total gaze paresis is present. Able to move one or both eyes, but may not be able to cross midline. 2 = Forced deviation. Total gaze paresis is not overcome by the oculocephalic maneuver.
3. Best Visual	0 = No visual loss. 1 = Partial hemianopia. Includes loss in only one quadrant. 2 = Complete hemianopia. Loss of vision in both top and bottom quadrants on the right or left side of a patient's visual field. 3 = Bilateral hemianopia. Blindness of any cause, including cortical blindness, or if visual loss is noted on both right and left sides of the visual fields.
4. Facial Palsy	0 = Normal. Symmetrical movements. 1 = Minor paralysis. Flattened nasolabial fold, asymmetry on smiling. 2 = Partial paralysis. Total or near-total paralysis of lower face. 3 = Complete paralysis of one or both sides of face. Absence of movement in the upper and lower face.
5. Motor Arm (a. Left Arm, b. Right Arm)	0 = No drift. Limb holds 90 (or 45) degrees for a full 10 seconds. 1 = Drift. Limb holds 90 (or 45) degrees, but then drifts down before full 10 seconds; does not hit bed or other support. 2 = Some effort against gravity. Limb cannot get to or maintain 90 (or 45) degrees, drifts down to bed, but has some effort against gravity. 3 = No effort against gravity. Limb falls. 4 = No movements. Flaccid extremities with no effort noted.
6. Motor Leg (a. Left Leg, b. Right Leg)	0 = No drift. Leg holds 30 degrees position for full five seconds. 1 = Drift. Leg falls by the end of the five second period, but does not hit bed. 2 = Some effort against gravity. Leg falls to bed by five seconds, but has some effort against gravity. 3 = No effort against gravity. Leg falls to bed immediately. 4 = No movement. Flaccid extremities with no effort noted.
7. Limb Ataxia	0 = Absent. 1 = Present in one limb. 2 = Present in two limbs.
8. Sensory	0 = Normal. No sensory loss. 1 = Mild to moderate sensory loss. Patient feels pin prick is less sharp or is dull on the affected side or there is a loss of superficial pain with pin prick, but patient is aware of being touched. 2 = Severe to total sensory loss. Patient is not aware of being touched on the face, arm and leg.
9. Best Language	0 = No aphasia. Normal fluent speech. 1 = Mild to moderate aphasia. Some obvious loss of fluency or facility of comprehension without significant limitation on ideas expressed or form of expression. Reduction of speech and/or comprehension however, makes conversation about provided materials difficult or impossible. For example, in conversation about provided materials, examiner can identify picture or naming card content from patient's response.

Table 2.1 (*continued*)

Description	Score
	2 = Severe aphasia. All communication is through fragmentary expression; great need for inference, questioning and guessing by the listener. Often limited to one-word answers. Range of information that can be exchanged is limited; listener carries burden of communication. Examiner cannot identify materials provided from patient response. 3 = Mute. Global aphasia. No usable speech or auditory comprehension.
10. Dysarthria	0 = Normal 1 = Mild to moderate dysarthria. Patient slurs at least some words and at worst, can be understood with some difficulty. 2 = Severe dysarthria. Patient's speech is so slurred as to be unintelligible in the absence of or out of proportion to any dysphasia or is nil (mute patient).
11. Extinction and Inattention (formerly neglect)	0 = Normal 1 = Visual, tactile, auditory, special or personal inattention or extinction to bilateral simultaneous stimulation in one of the sensory modalities. 2 = Profound hemi-inattention or extinction to more than one modality. Patient does not recognize own hand or orients to only one side of space.

corresponding to the middle cerebral artery (MCA) indicates presence of thrombus or embolus. Hypodensity in the basal ganglia, loss of differentiation between white and gray matter, and effacement of both the insular cortex and cortical gyri are early signs of ischemia. The presence of these signs affecting a large area of brain tissue is also associated with an increased risk of hemorrhagic transformation after the use of thrombolytic agents, especially when the area is larger than one third of MCA territory.[12]

Detection of these early signs may increase in sensitivity with the use of standard NCCT evaluation scores such as the Alberta Stroke Program Early CT Score (ASPECTS).[13] Changing the NCCT window on the workstation to show the difference between normal and abnormal brain tissue[14] is also helpful.

The diffusion-weighted sequences on Magnetic Resonance Imaging (MRI) of the brain are more sensitive than NCCT for stroke diagnosis as they identify the ischemic area as early as 35 minutes after the onset of symptoms. This method is especially useful when stroke diagnosis is uncertain. The ischemic area that appears in diffusion-weighted imaging corresponds approximately to the core infarct area in the brain.[15]

Several MRI protocols in SCs use diffusion-weighted and perfusion sequences to evaluate patients with an indeterminate therapeutic window or outside the therapeutic window, by defining in each patient the presence of viable brain tissue (penumbra). The hypothesis that supports this practice is that each individual has his own therapeutic window, based on his physiological tolerance to ischemia and the characteristics of the collateral arterial circulation of his brain. Vascular imaging with either arterial angioCT or angioMRI helps to locate the exact point of flow obstruction and is strongly recommended for endovascular reperfusion (in proximal occlusions of the anterior circulation, for example).[11] Choosing between these two imaging modalities depends on equipment availability and patient characteristics.

Transcranial Doppler (TCD) can be used to diagnose major cerebral artery occlusions and to monitor the effects of thrombolytic therapy; it also helps to determine the prognosis.[16,17] However, between 7 and 20% of patients with acute stroke do not have an adequate bone window; as a consequence, the scan cannot be performed.

Although brain NCCT has relatively low sensitivity in detecting small acute infarctions, especially in the posterior fossa, it is still the first choice in most centers that use thrombolytic therapy. For evaluation in the acute phase, it is sufficient, rapid, and available in most emergency departments; it can determine the presence of intracranial hemorrhage, and may also give prognostic information (early infarction signs). In patients who are candidates for thrombolytic therapy, NCCT should be performed within 25 minutes after the arrival at the emergency room, and the report should be obtained within the next 20 minutes.[9]

Supportive Care

Maintaining adequate Blood Pressure (BP) and oxygen saturation (≥ 92%), keeping body temperature lower than 37.5 °C and striving for euglycemia are the most important supportive therapies in the management of acute stroke. Continuous cardiac monitoring is recommended to detect early electrocardiographic signs of ischemia or arrhythmias.

In patients who are candidates for IV thrombolysis, treatment with rtPA should not be initiated if, at the time of administration, the patient has a BP of ≥ 185/110 mmHg.[9] This blood pressure reading should be decreased rapidly with IV drugs prior to the initiation of rtPA. Labetalol, nicardipine, esmolol or even sodium nitroprusside (if none of the first are available) are safe options. BP should be monitored before, during and after rtPA use. If the patient develops hypotension with antihypertensive treatment, decrease the dose and start infusion of physiological solution. Avoid infusion of solutions containing glucose to restore volume on account of the risk of dilutional hyponatremia.[9]

Studies of Intravenous Thrombolysis Use

Three clinical trials tested the use of streptokinase in the acute treatment of stroke and were early discontinued because of increased mortality and high rates of intracerebral hemorrhage.[17]

The use of rtPA in ischemic stroke up to 3 hours after the onset of symptoms was approved following the clinical trial of the National Institute of Neurological Diseases and Stroke (NINDS study, class I, evidence level A). The rtPA- treated group (dosage: 0.9 mg/kg) had 31% more patients with minimal or no neurological deficit at the assessment done three months after the stroke. There was a higher rate of symptomatic intracerebral hemorrhage in the treated group (6.4% x 0.6%, p < 0.001) but no increase in mortality (17% in the rtPA group x 21% in placebo). The benefit was demonstrated in all subtypes of stroke and was not affected by factors such as gender or age.

A meta-analysis of 6 studies with rtPA (2775 patients),[18] analyzed the outcome of patients treated between 0 and 6 hours after the onset of stroke. The results showed that the earlier the administration of rtPA, the better the outcome. The group treated up to 90 minutes after symptom onset had odds of 2.8 for a favorable outcome. Treatment between 181–270 minutes also had benefit (odds ratio 1.4). No benefit was observed among patients treated between 271–360 minutes. The bleeding rate in the rtPA group was 5.9% x 1.1% in the placebo group (p < 0.0001). In 2008, the benefit of IV rtPA use up to 4.5 hours after symptom onset was confirmed in the European Cooperative Acute Stroke Study III (ECASS III) trial,[4] extending the therapeutic window (class I, evidence level A). Several cohort studies performed after approval of rtPA confirmed the effectiveness of treatment with similar results to those of the NINDS study.[19]

The IST-3 (Third International Stroke Trial) study,[20] published in 2012, randomized patients with ischemic stroke to receive IV rtPA versus placebo up to 6 hours after symptom onset, selected by NCCT. A population outside the formal indication for treatment (elderly and with high baseline NIHSS score) was included; out of the 3035 study patients, 1617 (53%) were over 80 years of age. At 6 months the mortality rate was similar in both groups (26.9% on rtPA versus 26.7% on placebo). There was an increased risk of fatal and nonfatal hemorrhagic transformation with rtPA of 5.8%, as had been demonstrated in previous studies. The Oxford Handicap Score (OHS) assessment of independence after stroke did not differ significantly in the two groups (37% versus 35%). Therefore, there was no benefit with the use of rtPA in ischemic stroke up to 6 hours after symptom onset. The effect of treatment on patients over 80 years-old was at least as good as for those under that age.

In 2012, another meta-analysis[21] of 12 studies evaluated 7012 patients who received rtPA versus conventional treatment within 6 hours of the stroke onset. There was no difference in mortality between the groups at 3 months. There was a reduction in the composite outcome of death and severe functional disability of 4% (ARR = 4%, 95% CI 1.7–6%), benefiting 1 in every 25 patients treated at the 3-month assessment (NNT = 25 with 95% CI 16–59). The benefits were more expressive in patients treated up to 3 hours, with 1 in 11 treated patients becoming functionally independent – modified Rankin Score (mRS) 0 to 2 (RRA = 0.9%, 95% CI 0.46–1.34 and NNT = 11 with 95% CI 7–22) and 1 in 19 achieving minimal or no disability at 3 months - mRS 0 to 1 (RRA = 5.4% with 95% CI 3.2–7.6 for NNT = 19 with 95% CI 13–31). When comparing the subgroup of patients over 80 years old to those below that age, who received thrombolysis up to 3 hours after ischemic stroke onset, the use of rtPA brought benefit to both groups, allowing survival and/or functional independence in 20.7%, benefiting 1 out of 5 treated patients (ARR = 20.7%, 95% CI 14.4–27.0 with NNT = 5, 95% CI 4–7). Despite this being a subgroup analysis, the statistical power was 98.1%. In the same population, receiving rtPA within 6 hours of symptom onset, there is survival and/or independence benefit in 25.3%, which means increasing the survival or independence of 1 in 4 treated patients (ARR = 25.3%; 95% CI 21.8–28.8 and NNT = 4, 95% CI 3–5). The IST3 Study demonstrated that patients with NIHSS above 25 also benefit from EV thrombolysis.

Another important study of thrombolysis in stroke was published in 2016: the ENCHANTED study (Enhanced Control of Hypertension and Thrombolysis Stroke Study),[22] which compared the conventional dose of rtPA (0.9 mg kg EV) to the low dose (0.6 mg/ kg) in patients treated up to 4.5 hours after symptom onset. The objective was to evaluate whether the low dose was non-inferior to the conventional dose in achieving minimum or no disability at 3 months (Rankin modified between 0 and 1) and if the lower dose was safer (lower rate of symptomatic intracerebral hemorrhage). As a result, the lower dose did not reach non-inferiority at the primary endpoint, with 47% of patients achieving mRS 0–1 at 3 months when treated at low dose compared to 49% of patients receiving the standard dose, although it was assessed by shift analysis. In improving 1 point in the Rankin score at 3 months, the lower dose was not inferior to the standard dose (p = 0.04). In addition, the lower dose had lower rate of symptomatic intracranial hemorrhage and lower mortality related to the bleeding. The clinical relevance of the study is that the lower dose may be a therapeutic option in patients at higher risk of bleeding.

The main complication of thrombolytic treatment in stroke is symptomatic intracranial hemorrhage (sICH). The factors that most strongly predict the chance of bleeding after rtPA are: brain CT scan hypodensity in over 1/3 of the territory of the MCA (odds ratio 9.38), age above 75 years, BP above 180/105 mmHg at the start of rtPA infusion, diabetes (odds ratio of 2.69) and NIHSS of more than 20.[2,12,23] Despite the increased risk of bleeding, there is no upper age limit for treatment and elderly patients should not be excluded by this criterion alone. In addition to the risk of sICH, other potential adverse effects of medication include systemic bleeding, myocardial rupture in patients with recent transmural acute myocardial infarction, and anaphylactic reaction or angioedema secondary to rtPA, but these events are rare.[24] Orolingual angioedema (edema of the tongue, lips, or oropharynx) occurs in 1.3 to 5% of all patients receiving IV rtPA as treatment for ischemic stroke. Edema is typically mild, transient, and contralateral to the hemisphere of ischemic stroke and is generally associated with both previous use of angiotensin-converting enzyme inhibitor and infarcts involving the insular and frontal cortex. Recommendations for empirical treatment include IV ranitidine, diphenhydramine and methylprednisolone.

Although the efficacy of IV thrombolytic therapy in stroke has been well demonstrated, not all patients achieve vessel recanalization and some have initial recanalization with subsequent reocclusion. The rates of partial or complete recanalization of occlusion in the internal carotid artery are 10% and of the proximal occlusion in the MCA are 25–30%.[25,26] In addition, IV thrombolysis has a narrow therapeutic window and, due to its systemic effects, is contraindicated in many potential candidates[9]: patients with recent ischemic stroke, previous intracranial hemorrhage, recent head trauma, recent surgery or bleeding diathesis.

In an attempt to increase the rates of recanalization and, consequently, improve patient outcomes, endovascular reperfusion has been used in patients with large vessel occlusion. Anyway, IV thrombolysis is more easily implemented (it can be used in medium complexity hospitals without a hemodynamics unit) and, according to current evidence and international guidelines,[27,28] it should be used in eligible patients up to 4,5 hours after symptom onset, even with large vessel occlusion and endovascular treatment available, while endovascular treatment may be used in patients who fail to undergo IV treatment or in those who are ineligible for IV treatment up to 6 hours from symptom onset.

Treatment Recommendations for IV rtPA[9,10]

The protocol must be followed strictly in order to guarantee the safety of acute stroke treatment with IV thrombolysis:

Inclusion Criteria

a) Ischemic stroke in any cerebrovascular territory;
b) Possibility of initiating rtPA infusion within 4 hours and 30 minutes after symptom onset (which requires precise determination of symptom onset). If symptoms are noted on waking, the last time at which the patient was observed to be normal should be used instead;
c) No evidence of intracranial hemorrhage on head computed tomography (CT) scan or magnetic resonance imaging (MRI);
d) Age > 18 years.

Exclusion Criteria

a) Use of oral anticoagulants and prothrombin time (PT) > 15 s (INR > 1.7);

b) Use of heparin in the last 48 hours and prolonged aPTT;

c) History of ischemic stroke or severe head trauma in the last 3 months;

d) History of intracranial hemorrhage or cerebrovascular malformation;

e) Hypodensity of more than one-third of the middle cerebral artery territory on head CT;

f) Systolic blood pressure (SBP) ≤ 185 mmHg or diastolic blood pressure (DBP) ≤ 110 mmHg (on 3 separate measurements obtained at 10-minute intervals) refractory to antihypertensive agents;

g) Rapid and complete resolution of signs and symptoms before thrombolytic agent administration;

h) Mild neurological deficit (with no significant functional deterioration);

i) History of major surgery or invasive procedure in the last 2 weeks;

j) History of genitourinary or gastrointestinal bleeding in the last 3 weeks, or history of esophageal varices;

k) Arterial puncture at a non-compressible site within the last 7 days;

l) Coagulopathy (prolonged PT [INR > 1.7], prolonged aPTT, or platelet count < 100,000/mm3);

m) Blood glucose < 50 mg/dL with resolution of symptoms after hypoglycemia was treated;

n) Evidence of endocarditis, septic embolus, or pregnancy;

o) Recent myocardial infarction (occurring in the last 3 months) – a relative contra-indication;

p) Clinical suspicion of subarachnoid hemorrhage or acute aortic dissection.

Some centers use multimodal neuroimaging (MRI with diffusion and perfusion imaging or perfusion CT scan) to select candidates for thrombolytic therapy, particularly in patients outside the therapeutic window or when the exact time of symptom onset cannot be determined.

In patients with no recent history of oral anticoagulant or heparin use, rtPA infusion may be initiated before the results of a coagulation panel are available, but it should be discontinued if these results reveal an INR above 1.7, a prolonged aPTT as defined by local reference ranges, or a platelet count less than 100.000/mm3.

Acute Stroke Treatment Regimen with IV rtPA

a) Transfer the patient to the Intensive Care Unit or to the acute Stroke Unit;

b) Initiate intravenous rtPA infusion 0.9 mg/kg giving 10% bolus in 1 minute and the remainder in 1 hour. Do not exceed the maximum dose of 90 mg. There is the option of using the dose of 0.6 mg (15% bolus and the remainder within 1 hour) for those patients at higher risk of bleeding;

c) Do not give heparin, antiplatelet therapy or anticoagulant within the first 24 hours of thrombolytic use;

d) Do not feed the patient for 24 hours due to the risk of hemorrhagic transformation and the need for urgent surgical intervention;

e) Repeat the neurological examination (NIHSS score) every 15 minutes during infusion, every 30 minutes in the next 6 hours, and thereafter every hour until 24 hours;

f) Monitor BP every 15 minutes in the first 2 hours, every 30 minutes in the next 6 hours of treatment;

g) If the BP is above 180/105 mmHg: initiate labetalol, nicardipine or intravenous esmolol and maintain SBP < 180 mmHg. Alternative: sodium nitroprusside (0.5 mg/kg/min);

h) Monitor BP every 15 minutes during antihypertensive treatment. Beware of the risk of hypotension;

i) If there is any suspicion of intracranial hemorrhage, suspend rtPA and request an urgent brain NCCT, blood count, PT, aPTT, platelet count and fibrinogen;

j) Repeat brain NCCT in 24 hours after thrombolysis to evaluate complications;

k) After 24 hours of thrombolytic treatment (and after ruling out hemorrhage on the NCCT), stroke treatment follows the same guidelines on antiplatelet or anticoagulation as in the patient who did not receive thrombolysis

2.1.2 Patient Follow-up and Timing Goals

The functional outcome of post-stroke patients is generally measured by the modified Rankin Scale (mRS) at 3 months (▶ Table 2.2). The most frequent outcome for good evolution in IV thrombolysis is mRS 0–1 at 3 months (minimum or no disability).

Table 2.2 Post-stroke functional assessment scale-modified Rankin scale

Score		Description
0	No symptoms at all	
1	No significant disability despite symptoms	able to carry out all usual duties and activities
2	Slight disability	unable to carry out all previous activities, but able to look after own affairs without assistance
3	Moderate disability	requiring some help, but able to walk without assistance
4	Moderately severe disability	unable to walk without assistance and unable to attend to own bodily needs without assistance
5	Severe disability	bedridden, incontinent and requiring constant nursing care and attention
6	Dead	

Table 2.3 Timing goal for acute stroke in the emergency

	Time limit
Door-to-physician	≥ 10 min
Door-to-neurologist	≥ 15 min
Door-to-CT	≥ 25 min
Door-to-needle (> 80% of compliance)	≥ 60 min

For proper functioning of a stroke center (SC), the results should be measured and monitored frequently in order to solve any issues. In addition to the functional results, it is important to measure the recommended timing goals for SCs (► Table 2.3), seeking to reduce them continuously so that the treatment is more rapidly initiated, which increases the benefit for the patients.

2.2 Stroke Centers and Stroke Units

Besides the major individual impact of reperfusion therapy, the Stroke Unit (SU) is the intervention with the greatest population impact that benefits all stroke patients.[29]

The SU is the key point of the entire stroke care delivery and it works integrating all specialists of the SU team, emergency and other hospital areas, with outside specialists and primary care physicians. It is fundamental for the training and the teaching of specialists who are responsible for the care of these patients, thereby helping the local organization of the Stroke Network.[30]

The principal models of SCs and SUs will be discussed here: their fundamental components, their impact and the implementation models in Brazil and other countries.

First of all, it is important to distinguish between SC and SU.[23,29] The SCs are hospitals ready to treat stroke patients with a trained and specialized multidisciplinary team, provided with all the necessary technology to offer the best evidence-based treatment. These SCs may or may not have a SU. The SU is a physically defined area with exclusive beds for stroke patients assisted by an interdisciplinary trained team, specialized in the hospital treatment of these patients.[29] Rather than high technology, the main feature of these SUs is the systematic approach of care, which is affordable even in low-complexity hospitals. The most important component is the team, which works with definite objectives: taking the stroke patient to the best possible level of functionality, educating the patient and the family for post-stroke care and preparing them to manage the difficulties. The implementation of a SU decreases mortality in stroke patients by 17% and dependency by 25%.[29,31,32]

The Stroke Care Network dates to the emergence of SUs in Scandinavian countries in the 1980s, a model that spread initially throughout Europe. In 1995, the Helsingborg Declaration under the motto "Stroke Units for All" sought to improve stroke management in European countries by unifying and standardizing stroke care. This action was able to reduce mortality by 20% and achieve functional independence by 70% in the first three months.[33] Since then, in parallel with managers perceiving local challenges regarding attendance and follow-up of the stroke patient, the SUs were disseminated. The need to reduce the time for diagnosis and initiation of reperfusion therapies followed, which took stroke care closer to the patient – from Telemedicine to brain CT and IV thrombolysis inside the ambulance, in the Mobile Units/Stroke Mobile Teams (► Fig. 2.1).

2.2.1 Stroke Centers

The concept of SC[23] originated in the United States and Canada. The Comprehensive Stroke Center (CSC), a tertiary level facility with a high flow of patients, provides acute stroke care by specialized neurologists supported by advanced neuroimaging, neurointervention and neurosurgery techniques as

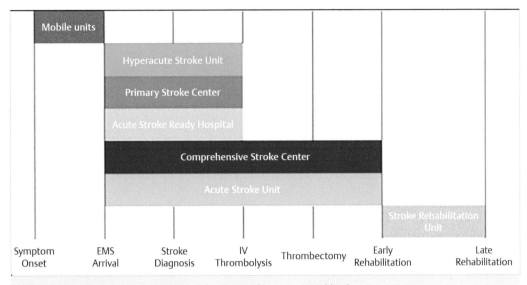

Fig. 2.1 Types of Stroke Care Services and the phases of care comprised by them.

well as intensive care units. The CSC can be structured to receive patients directly from pre-hospital services or patients referred by Primary Stroke Centers (PSC) and Acute Stroke Ready Hospitals (ASRH).

The PSC are units with emergency physicians or neurologists trained in stroke care, with tomography available 24 hours a day, 7 days a week, and basic structure for stroke care - they must perform reperfusion treatment (at least with IV thrombolysis) and have access to the neurointensive care unit.

The ASRH is a term applied to any hospital with acute stroke care infrastructure, including rapid thrombolytic therapy (door-to-needle time under 60 minutes). The center should be able to diagnose, stabilize, and refer the patient to a PSC or CSC.

2.2.2 Stroke Units

Types of Stroke Units

Acute Stroke Unit

The Acute SU was created to enable acute phase stroke treatment. It admits patients in the hyperacute phase (first hours of stroke), with an average hospitalization of 5 days, allowing a more strict control of the physiological variables and early mobilization. Most cases need no referral to Intensive Care Units (ICU).[23,29,31]

Rehabilitation Stroke Unit

The Rehabilitation SU receives the patient after the acute phase and stabilization. Hospitalization is prolonged: weeks to months. The interdisciplinary team works on the rehabilitation and education of the patient and his family.[23,29,31]

Integrated Stroke Units (Comprehensive Stroke Unit)

The Comprehensive Stroke Unit, staffed by a complete interdisciplinary team and equipped with monitored beds, admits the patient in the hyperacute phase, provides acute phase treatment and initiates early rehabilitation. The average length of stay is 14 days. According to the literature, this model, which promotes continuity in care, offers the greatest benefit.[23,29,31]

These Units are called High Complexity Units of Stroke, Comprehensive Stroke Units in Europe or Integrated Stroke Units in Canada. This care can be offered in the same facility or in separate facilities, as in the case of the German model - acute phase care, etiological definition and early rehabilitation occur in one location, and subsequent continuing rehabilitation occurs in another, by distinct teams.

Impact

Meta-analysis of randomized clinical trials demonstrate that SU care is effective in reducing the relative risk of death in one year by 13% (95% CI 0.69 to 0.94, p = 0.005), dependence or death in 21% (95% CI 0.68 to 0.90, p = 0.0007) and death or institutionalization in 22% (95% CI 0.68 to 0.89, p = 0.0003).[31,32]

These outcomes are achieved because of reduced immobility-related complications (deep venous thrombosis, aspiration pneumonia, urinary tract infection).[32] Patients in SU were more often monitored and received more oxygen therapy and antipyretics; they were evaluated for dysphagia earlier, in order to reduce aspiration-associated pneumonia, and they also benefited from early nutritional support, with fewer cases of stroke progression, respiratory infection or dehydration.[34] All subgroups of patients presented benefit regardless of gender, age or severity of Stroke.[31,32,34,35]

The SU has been shown to be both clinically effective and cost-effective, the main gain being life years saved.[31,32,34,35] The benefit of SU was also verified in the real world setting.[36,37,38,39,40] Out of 41,692 patients in Scotland[40] in routine care, 79% of patients were treated in SU and 21% in general units. The chance of being alive in 7 days was 3 times higher in the group treated in SU (95% CI 2.71 to 3.56) and in 1 year was 1.43 times higher (95% CI 1.34 to 1.54), while the Odds Ratio for home discharge (without institutionalization) was 1.19 times higher (95% CI 1.11 to 1.28).

Number of Beds

The recommended number of beds in SU is 10 beds for every 200,000 inhabitants for a given area (or 20 beds for every 800 cases of stroke).[30]

Team

The SU team depends on the type of Unit. Here is the recommended team[41] composition for the Comprehensive Stroke Units: Neurologist (Stroke specialist - coordinator), Neurologist or physician with specialization in Stroke, Nurse (1 coordinator), Nursing Assistant (1 per 6 hours-shift), Nursing technicians, Physical Therapist, Occupational Therapist, Pharmacist, Speech Therapist (focusing on dysphagia), Social Worker, Nutritionist, Psychologist, Neurosurgeon, Vascular Surgeon, Neuroradiologist.

Essential Structure

The WSO published in 2014 the Global Stroke Services Guidelines,[42] focusing on low and middle income countries and making recommendations on the maximum desired structure for stroke services, a minimum essential framework for stroke services, and the suitable care in places that have little access to physicians and health professionals (the least that should be done for the stroke care). The essential structure for an organized SU[41,42] in addition to exclusive beds for stroke patients, should have at least the following staff:
- A neurologist (preferably a neurologist specialized in Stroke) as team coordinator and, if the acute treatment is performed at a SU, a physician 24 hours a day;
- 24-hour of Nursing care (by a nurse trained in stroke care);
- Nursing technician (ideally at least 1 every 4 beds);
- Daily Physical Therapist support;
- Daily Speech Therapist support (if not possible, a nursing technician should be trained to assess dysphagia);
- Neurologist supporting the team coordinator, twenty-four hours a day, seven days a week (face-to-face, on-call or by telemedicine).

The SU must have at least the following material resources:
- At least two equipments for continuous and controlled infusion of fluids ("infusion pump") for each bed, with an operational reserve of one equipment every three beds;
- Wall connections for oxygen, as well as station outlets for medical compressed air with pressure regulators and medical vacuum for each bed;
- Materials for aspiration;
- Equipment for measuring blood glucose;
- Transportable oxygen cylinder;
- A face mask with different oxygen concentrations for every three beds
- Equipment for blood pressure measurement;
- In the acute SU, a bedside monitor for continuous monitoring of heart rate, electrocardiography, pulse oxymetry, non-invasive pressure, respiratory rate and temperature, for each bed.

The hospital should have at least:
- Brain CT scan (the benefit of SU is evident even in hospitals without CT, but it increases greatly with the use of CT);
- Equipment for Electrocardiogram (ECG);
- Laboratory service;
- Minimum structure to investigate the etiology of stroke: transthoracic Doppler echocardiography, carotid Doppler ultrasound;
- Ideally, local access to brain MRI (or assistance agreement within the Network), angiotomography or angioresonance of

intracranial and extracranial vessels, transcranial Doppler, transesophageal echocardiogram, and digital angiography.

2.2.3 Quality Indicators of Care

It is essential to measure quality indicators of care so that failures are recognized and the unit subsequently restructured and retrained according to the results. At least the following indicators should be monitored[30,42,43]:

- Prophylaxis for deep venous thrombosis initiated by the second day;
- Hospital discharge on an antiplatelet drug in patients with non-cardioembolic ischemic stroke;
- Hospital discharge on oral anticoagulation for patients with ischemic stroke and atrial fibrillation (AF) or "flutter", except for contraindications;
- Use of antiplatelet agents in patients with ischemic stroke, started up to the second day of hospitalization;
- Hospital discharge on statin for patients with atherothrombotic stroke;
- Hospital discharge with a prophylactic and rehabilitation therapy plan;
- Percentage of patients with acute cerebrovascular disease treated in the SU;
- Length of hospital stay of the patient affected by stroke aiming to reduce it;
- Monitoring of the following complications, aiming to reduce them: deep venous thrombosis, pressure ulcers, pneumonia, urinary tract infection;
- Hospital mortality due to stroke, aiming to reduce it;
- Door-to-tomography time below 25 minutes;
- Door-to-needle time below 60 minutes.

2.2.4 Stroke Centers in the World

Developing Countries (Low and Middle Income Countries)

The particularities of several countries regarding stroke care will be discussed below. Understanding these differences can help establish priorities to achieve the goal of providing consistent evidence-based care regardless of location.

Brazil

In Brazil,[10] 100% of the population is entitled to free health care, funded by the Federal Government.

Only 20% of the population has additional private health insurance. The National Pre-hospital is called SAMU and its call number is 192. It covers 70% of the population.

Stroke care in Brazil has changed substantially in recent years.[10] After the publication of Ordinance 665, dated April 2012,[3] in the Official Journal of the Brazilian Government, the criteria for the accreditation of SCs in Brazil were established and structured according to available resources and the real conditions of the hospitals in the country. The main component is the interdisciplinary team. This ordinance was revised in June 2015 as Ordinance 800.

In 2011, a free online training course for stroke care sponsored by several institutions (Neurology Society, Stroke Society, Brazilian Stroke Network and Brazilian Medical Association) was implemented for all health professionals at all levels (pre-hospital, hospital and primary care). The SCs work in pre-hospital networks, mostly in sites that are already organized. Despite major advances, less than 1% of stroke patients in the country receive thrombolysis (this number increases to 10–20% in stroke centers).

Three types of hospitals were established: Urgent Care Centers Type I, II and III.

Urgent Care Centers Type I

These referral hospitals for stroke care provide and perform IV thrombolysis as treatment and have a minimum structure for stroke care. These hospitals do not have a SU and must meet the following requirements: perform emergency care 24 hours a day; perform brain CT scan 24 hours a day; to have a team trained in emergency care for stroke patients, consisting of a physician, nurse, and nursing technicians, this team being coordinated by a clinical neurologist; to provide written clinical and care protocols; to provide neurological care coverage, available within 30 minutes of patient admission (continuous ward duty or on call - or specialized neurological support through telemedicine); to have monitored beds for acute stroke care, with a physician 24 hours a day and staff trained to that effect; to perform full-time clinical laboratory service; to have a twenty-four hours neurosurgical team (face-to-face or available in up to two hours) and hemotherapy service.

Telemedicine for acute stroke treatment consists of teleconferencing systems that include the sharing of video, sound and neuroimaging data, all of which permits remote assessment of a patient suspected of stroke by a neurologist experienced in stroke, preferably linked to a Stroke Reference Center. In this evaluation, the system must allow this neurologist to perform a check of the patient's clinical history and neurological examination and to evaluate the neuroimaging performed in the remote equipment in real time.

Urgent Care Centers Type II

These referral hospital establishments for stroke care must meet all the requirements for the Type I Center and have an acute SU as well. They should:
a) have a definite physical area with at least five beds exclusively for the care of acute stroke (either ischemic, hemorrhagic or transient ischemic attack), coordinated by a neurologist;
b) perform care for the acute stroke patient up to 72 hours of hospitalization, offering IV thrombolysis for ischemic stroke;
c) perform multiprofessional care, including physical therapy and speech therapy;
d) ensure that the acute phase treatment is coordinated by a neurologist;
e) perform the following procedures: ECG, full-time clinical laboratory service, radiology service;
f) have access, on the spot or in another facility, to: Doppler ultrasonography of cervical vessels, transthoracic and transesophageal echocardiography, angiography, MRI, angioCT or angioMRI, transcranial Doppler and interventional neuroradiology.

Urgent Care Centers Type III to Stroke Patients

These are hospital establishments that meet all the requirements for Centers type I and II, also have an Integral SU, which includes the Stroke Acute Care Unit (they may share the same physical space or not), and meet the following requirements:
a) at least ten beds;
b) coordination by a neurologist, dedicated to the care of patients affected by stroke (either ischemic, hemorrhagic or transient ischemic attack), up to 15 days of hospitalization;
c) ability to take care of all acute stroke cases admitted to the institution, except those requiring intensive care and those who only need supportive palliative care;
d) treatment of the acute phase, early rehabilitation and complete etiological investigation;
e) specialized outpatient clinic.

The Integral SU must have the following features:
a) 1 neurologist as coordinator;
b) 1 physician, 24 hours a day;
c) neurologist as support, 24 hours a day;
d) 1 nurse in the unit;
e) 1 nursing technician every four beds;
f) 1 physical therapist every ten beds, six hours a day;
g) 1 speech therapist every ten beds, six hours a day;
h) 1 occupational therapist every ten beds, six hours a day;
i) 1 social worker, 6 hours a day, from Monday to Friday;
j) supportive care by psychologist, nutritionist and pharmacist in the institution;

Currently, Brazil has 149 Stroke Centers (public and private), 49% with SU and, out of the total, 51 are licensed by the Ministry of Health.

Chile

The Chilean Ministry of Health has a National Stroke Plan and National Guidelines for stroke care.[44] The population is taken care of by the Public System in 80% of cases, the remaining 20% has additional health insurance. There is still a lack of awareness of stroke warning signs and prevention. IV thrombolysis was implemented a few years ago in private facilities and in recent years also in the public health system. Thrombectomy is available in public and private facilities. Public hospitals (SCs), which perform at least 50 thrombolysis per year, receive reimbursement for endovascular treatment as well. In the beginning of 2017, the country had 16 public CSC, 12 private and 4 military. In 2016 a telemedicine service was implemented in Santiago, as well as an online stroke training course for all health professionals (offered by the Ministry of Health).

Argentina

The country has established a National Registry of Stroke (Argentinian National Stroke Registry [ReNACer]),[45] funded by the Ministry of Health. Data from this registry show that 79% of patients received antithrombotic therapy within 48 hours of admission to a SU. However, the number of patients treated with thrombolysis in the SU is still low (5.7%). Treatment also varies whether the patient is admitted to an academic hospital or not. In university hospitals, the mortality rate is lower

(7.1%) compared to non-university hospitals (10.6%). But even considering only university hospitals, the admission rate in SUs is still low (5.7%). A positive aspect is a short hospitalization time (5 days). About 90.2% of patients with ischemic stroke are discharged on antithrombotic therapy. The SUs are in the process of settling down in the country, including recent experiences with Mobile Stroke Units. In addition to the low number of SUs, the country faces another limitation which is an insufficient number of specialists prepared to act in the cerebrovascular area as compared to the size of the population.[46]

Mexico

The first SUs were inaugurated in 2010, and the country has encountered challenges to maintain these centers.[47] Currently, the country invests in education, prevention, and both medical and paramedical care. One of the limitations in treating stroke is the ability of the population to recognize signs of the ongoing disease. Assessments showed that only 37% of the population recognized an alarm symptom.[47] Less than 3% managed to name more than 3 signs of disease manifestation, demonstrating the need for investment in education. Despite these limitations, the country has carried out several initiatives. They carried out a door-to-door study to detail the epidemiology of the disease in the country.[48] In addition, they have representative data regarding the etiology of the disease that can help guide prevention policies.[49] Another bottleneck faced by the country is to reduce the number of patients with moderate to severe functional dependence, especially in rural areas, a situation that is apparently exacerbated by the fact that the country does not have universal health coverage.

China

Since the first SU in 2001, the country has become an example of how SUs can change the prognosis of stroke when it comes to developing countries. A previous study showed that the mortality reported at 28 and 120 days was substantially lower when the patient was under care of this type of specialized unit in China.[50] In addition, the average time spent in the SU is shorter (37 days) compared to hospital stay in a common ward unit (69 days). Interestingly, China has been noted not only for the heavy investment in treatment according to Western techniques, but also for trying to integrate the knowledge of Oriental Medicine for the benefit of the patient.[51]

India

India is another Asian giant that is trying to spread a stroke care program across a country presenting some barriers to diffusion, like territorial extension and regional cultural differences. Funding for stroke care programs, as in all other developing countries discussed here, is another big issue. The country has a shortage of trained professionals to deal with the patient's particularities in acute cerebrovascular disease, which emphasizes the need to attract non-neurological medical professionals to address this deficiency in a short- to medium-term.[52] There is also a clear concentration of SUs in urban university centers, a situation that certainly afflicts other developing countries. But through effective measures, the country has taken significant steps to better understand and treat the disease in its territory. Recently, the government of India has inaugurated the National Program for Prevention and Control of Cancer, Diabetes, Cardiovascular Diseases & Stroke (NPCDCS),[53] a clear incentive for activities of prevention and control of noncommunicable diseases.

Vietnam

Like other developing countries at present, Vietnam is experiencing a transition from infectious diseases to chronic diseases, and the country is trying to adapt quickly to this new reality. Vietnam does not have a specific medical association for the study of cerebrovascular disease, and the training of the professionals who will be in charge of the stroke care is distributed equally among the societies of Cardiology and Neurology. Investigation of the disease occurs primarily through hospital-based studies that do not represent community data.[54] The country has less than 10 SUs concentrated in the public administration, and a few in private facilities. The number of professionals trained in the care of these patients, regardless of the type of institution, is insufficient for the amount of work required. Often family members are recruited in order to provide care for which they have not been adequately trained and this can inflate the issue of hospital-associated infection.[54] Public understanding of the need for urgent care is also limited, and many resort to methods such as acupuncture for immediate care instead of turning to a specialized medical unit. Like SUs, rtPA treatment was introduced in the year 2000. But even now thrombolytic treatment is reserved for a few units in Vietnam. The only hope of bringing more benefits to patients in the acute phase resides in the formation of new groups interested in changing the situation.

Developed Countries (High Income Countries)

Europe

In 1995, the Helsingborg Declaration standardized stroke care in Europe, reducing mortality and functional dependence. In the second edition of the Helsingborg Declaration, the main objectives in the management and stroke care were: continuous care from acute SU to rehabilitation and secondary prevention strategies. By 2015, the main goals were that more than 85% of patients survived the first month after stroke, that 70% of survivors remained independent in the third month, and that all patients with acute stroke were transferred to hospitals with adequate capacity and experience, defined as SUs or areas dedicated to stroke.[55]

Both establishment of SUs and adherence to European stroke guidelines have led to a significant reduction in mortality and disability regardless of age, gender and race.[32]

There are two distinct realities. In the countries of Central Eastern Europe there has been an increase in stroke rates and stroke-related deaths.[56] In Western European countries, even though the absolute number of strokes has increased due to population aging, the incidence has decreased in the last two decades.[57] Most likely, the organizational models of each site have influenced the different results obtained.

In Austria, three care levels in stroke centers were defined: CSC, PSC and a minimum level required for hospital wards that admit stroke patients. In addition, a management quality certification was implemented to check the performance of this system. Since 1990, a standardized model analyzes system performance. The results are assessed by the local authorities and are confidential. In 2008, the NQZ (Nationals Qualitätszertifikat) pilot program of voluntary certification for home caregivers was launched to assess internal management quality and performance of outcome-oriented indicators. The Austrian model was approved by the European Stroke Organization (ESO).

In Switzerland, according to the Swiss Stroke Society, a stroke management system is needed to adhere to ESO's recommendations for establishing SUs and SCs. In 2012, the IVHSM (Interkantonale Hochspezialisierten Vereinigung der Medizin) established the SFCNS (Swiss Federation Clinical-Neuro-Societies) -Hirnschlagkommission (HK), composed of neurology, internal medicine and intensive medicine societies. SFCNS-HK is committed to development of certification programs, formation of a certification body for SCs and SUs in accordance with national and international guidelines, and coordination of continuing stroke education.

The TEMPiS (Telemedical Project for Integrative Stroke Care) project, located in Bavaria (Germany), was one of the first Telestroke projects in Europe. In the first decade of the TEMPiS project, the proportion of patients with stroke and TIA admitted to hospitals with stroke units increased from 19–78%.[58]

2.3 Final Considerations

In addition to the organization of the SCs and, the SUs and the implementation of the reperfusion treatment, it is fundamental to organize the local systems of care and the stroke care delivery. It is important to agree with the local health authorities regarding the organization of the referral network in the region for a better distribution of patients through the pre-hospital rescue service (EMS). Furthermore, all stroke patients should be attended to and controlled by the EMS, whether they are at home, at the Primary Care Unit or at a hospital that is not a referral facility for stroke, and from there, they should be directed to the Stroke Center in the shortest possible time. The entire network should be trained in stroke care, including case detection, treatment and prevention. And, finally, stroke education must reach the population in order to be effective. This whole process, when implemented, results in an important reduction in the burden of stroke.

References

[1] Feigin VL, Mensah GA, Norrving B, Murray CJ, Roth GA, GBD 2013 Stroke Panel Experts Group. Atlas of the Global Burden of Stroke (1990–2013): The GBD 2013 Study. Neuroepidemiology. 2015; 45(3):230–236

[2] The National Institute of Neurological Disorders and Stroke rt-pa Stroke Study Group. Tissue plasminogen activator for acute ischemic stroke. N Engl J Med. 1995; 333:1581–1587

[3] Muñoz Venturelli P, Robinson T, Lavados PM, et al. HeadPoST Investigators. Regional variation in acute stroke care organisation. J Neurol Sci. 2016; 371:126–130

[4] Hacke W, Kaste M, Bluhmki E, et al. ECASS Investigators. Thrombolysis with alteplase 3 to 4.5 hours after acute ischemic stroke. N Engl J Med. 2008; 359(13):1317–1329

[5] Winkler DT, Fluri F, Fuhr P, et al. Thrombolysis in stroke mimics: frequency, clinical characteristics, and outcome. Stroke. 2009; 40(4):1522–1525

[6] Scott PA, Silbergleit R. Misdiagnosis of stroke in tissue plasminogen activator-treated patients: characteristics and outcomes. Ann Emerg Med. 2003; 42(5):611–618

[7] Chernyshev OY, Martin-Schild S, Albright KC, et al. Safety of tPA in stroke mimics and neuroimaging-negative cerebral ischemia. Neurology. 2010; 74(17):1340–1345

[8] Saver JL, Barsan WG. Swift or sure?: The acceptable rate of neurovascular mimics among IV tPA-treated patients. Neurology. 2010; 74(17):1336–1337

[9] Jauch EC, Saver JL, Adams HP, Jr, et al. American Heart Association Stroke Council, Council on Cardiovascular Nursing, Council on Peripheral Vascular Disease, Council on Clinical Cardiology. Guidelines for the early management of patients with acute ischemic stroke: a guideline for healthcare professionals from the American Heart Association/American Stroke Association. Stroke. 2013; 44(3):870–947

[10] Martins SC, Pontes-Neto OM, Alves CV, et al. Brazilian Stroke Network. Past, present, and future of stroke in middle-income countries: the Brazilian experience. Int J Stroke. 2013; 8 Suppl A100:106–111

[11] Saur D, Kucinski T, Grzyska U, et al. Sensitivity and interrater agreement of CT and diffusion-weighted MR imaging in hyperacute stroke. AJNR Am J Neuroradiol. 2003; 24(5):878–885

[12] Hacke W, Kaste M, Fieschi C, et al. The European Cooperative Acute Stroke Study (ECASS). Intravenous thrombolysis with recombinant tissue plasminogen activator for acute hemispheric stroke. JAMA. 1995; 274(13):1017–1025

[13] Barber PA, Demchuk AM, Zhang J, Buchan AM. Validity and reliability of a quantitative computed tomography score in predicting outcome of hyperacute stroke before thrombolytic therapy. ASPECTS Study Group. Alberta Stroke Programme Early CT Score. [published correction appears in Lancet. 2000;355:2170]. Lancet. 2000; 355(9216):1670–1674

[14] Lev MH, Farkas J, Gemmete JJ, et al. Acute stroke: improved nonenhanced CT detection–benefits of soft-copy interpretation by using variable window width and center level settings. Radiology. 1999; 213(1):150–155

[15] Demchuk AM, Burgin WS, Christou I, et al. Thrombolysis in brain ischemia (TIBI) transcranial Doppler flow grades predict clinical severity, early recovery, and mortality in patients treated with intravenous tissue plasminogen activator. Stroke. 2001; 32(1):89–93

[16] Alexandrov AV, Wojner AW, Grotta JC, CLOTBUST Investigators. CLOTBUST: design of a randomized trial of ultrasound-enhanced thrombolysis for acute ischemic stroke. J Neuroimaging. 2004; 14(2):108–112

[17] Adams HP, Jr, del Zoppo G, Alberts MJ, et al. American Heart Association, American Stroke Association Stroke Council, Clinical Cardiology Council, Cardiovascular Radiology and Intervention Council, Atherosclerotic Peripheral Vascular Disease and Quality of Care Outcomes in Research Interdisciplinary Working Groups. Guidelines for the early management of adults with ischemic stroke: a guideline from the American Heart Association/American Stroke Association Stroke Council, Clinical Cardiology Council, Cardiovascular Radiology and Intervention Council, and the Atherosclerotic Peripheral Vascular Disease and Quality of Care Outcomes in Research Interdisciplinary Working Groups: the American Academy of Neurology affirms the value of this guideline as

an educational tool for neurologists. Stroke. 2007; 38(5):1655–1711

[18] The ATLANTIS, ECASS, and NINDS rt-PA study group investigators. Association of outcome with early stroke treatment: Pooled analysis of ATLANTIS, ECASSs, and NINDS rt-PA stroke trials. Lancet. 2004; 363:768–774

[19] Wahlgren N, Ahmed N, Dávalos A, et al. SITS-MOST investigators. Thrombolysis with alteplase for acute ischaemic stroke in the Safe Implementation of Thrombolysis in Stroke-Monitoring Study (SITS-MOST): an observational study. Lancet. 2007; 369(9558):275–282

[20] Sandercock P, Wardlaw JM, Lindley RI, et al. IST-3 collaborative group. The benefits and harms of intravenous thrombolysis with recombinant tissue plasminogen activator within 6 h of acute ischaemic stroke (the third international stroke trial [IST-3]): a randomised controlled trial. Lancet. 2012; 379(9834):2352–2363

[21] Wardlaw JM, Murray V, Berge E, et al. Recombinant tissue plasminogen activator for acute ischaemic stroke: an updated systematic review and meta-analysis. Lancet. 2012; 379 (9834):2364–2372

[22] Anderson CS, Robinson T, Lindley RI, et al. ENCHANTED Investigators and Coordinators. Low-Dose versus Standard-Dose Intravenous Alteplase in Acute Ischemic Stroke. N Engl J Med. 2016; 374(24):2313–2323

[23] Theofanidis D, Savopoulos C, Hatzitolios A. Global specialized stroke care delivery models. J Vasc Nurs. 2016; 34(1):2–11

[24] Hill MD, Lye T, Moss H, et al. Hemi-orolingual angioedema and ACE inhibition after alteplase treatment of stroke. Neurology. 2003; 60(9):1525–1527

[25] Alexandrov AV, Molina CA, Grotta JC, et al. CLOTBUST Investigators. Ultrasound-enhanced systemic thrombolysis for acute ischemic stroke. N Engl J Med. 2004; 351(21):2170–2178

[26] Wolpert SM, Bruckmann H, Greenlee R, Wechsler L, Pessin MS, del Zoppo GJ. Neuroradiologic evaluation of patients with acute stroke treated with recombinant tissue plasminogen activator. The rt-PA Acute Stroke Study Group. AJNR Am J Neuroradiol. 1993; 14(1):3–13

[27] Powers WJ, Derdeyn CP, Biller J, et al. AHA/ASA Focused Update of the 2013 Guidelines for the Early Management of Patients With Acute Ischemic Stroke Regarding Endovascular Treatment. A guideline for healthcare professionals from the American Heart Association/American Stroke Association. Stroke. 2015; 2015:46

[28] Pontes-Neto OM, Cougo P, Martins SCO, et al. Brazilian guidelines for endovascular treatment of patients with acute ischemic stroke. Arq Neuropsiquiatr. 2017; 75(1):50–56

[29] Stroke Unit Trialists' Collaboration. Organised inpatient (stroke unit) care for stroke. In: Cochrane Library. Issue 1, 2007

[30] Portaria 665 de 12 de Abril de 2012 Diário Oficial da União. Ministério da saúde. Available at: http://portalsaude.saude. gov.br/index.php/o-ministerio/principal/secretarias/900-sas-raiz/daet-raiz/media-e-alta-complexidade/l5-media-e-alta-complexidade/12676-cgmac-teste-botao-14. Accessed in February 2017

[31] Collaborative systematic review of the randomised trials of organised inpatient (stroke unit) care after stroke. Stroke Unit Trialists' Collaboration. BMJ. 1997; 314(7088):1151–1159

[32] Stroke Unit Trialists' Collaboration. Organised inpatient (stroke unit) care for stroke. Cochrane Database Syst Rev. 2013; 9(9):CD000197

[33] Norrving B, International Society of Internal Medicine, European Stroke Council, International Stroke Society, WHO Regional Office for European. The 2006 Helsingborg consen-

sus on European Stroke Strategies: Summary of conference proceedings and background to the 2nd Helsingborg Declaration. Int J Stroke. 2007; 2(2):139–143

[34] Evans A, Perez I, Harraf F, et al. Can differences in management processes explain different outcomes between stroke unit and stroke-team care? Lancet. 2001; 358(9293):1586–1592

[35] Te Ao BJ, Brown PM, Feigin VL, Anderson CS. Are stroke units cost effective? Evidence from a New Zealand stroke incidence and population-based study. Int J Stroke. 2012; 7(8):623–630

[36] Seenan P, Long M, Langhorne P. Stroke units in their natural habitat: systematic review of observational studies. Stroke. 2007; 38(6):1886–1892

[37] Di Carlo A, Lamassa M, Wellwood I, et al. European Registers of Stroke (EROS) Project. Stroke unit care in clinical practice: an observational study in the Florence center of the European Registers of Stroke (EROS) Project. Eur J Neurol. 2011; 18(5):686–694

[38] Terént A, Asplund K, Farahmand B, et al. Riks-Stroke Collaboration. Stroke unit care revisited: who benefits the most? A cohort study of 105,043 patients in Riks-Stroke, the Swedish Stroke Register. J Neurol Neurosurg Psychiatry. 2009; 80(8): 881–887

[39] Candelise L, Gattinoni M, Bersano A, Micieli G, Sterzi R, Morabito A, PROSIT Study Group. Stroke-unit care for acute stroke patients: an observational follow-up study. Lancet. 2007; 369 (9558):299–305

[40] Turner M, Barber M, Dodds H, et al. The impact of stroke unit care on outcome in a Scottish stroke population, taking into account case mix and selection bias. J Neurol Neurosurg Psychiatry. 2014

[41] Langhorne P, Pollock A, Stroke Unit Trialists' Collaboration. What are the components of effective stroke unit care? Age Ageing. 2002; 31(5):365–371

[42] Lindsay P, Furie KL, Davis SM, Donnan GA, Norrving B. World Stroke Organization global stroke services guidelines and action plan. Int J Stroke. 2014; 9 Suppl A100:4–13

[43] Schwamm LH, Fonarow GC, Reeves MJ, et al. Get With the Guidelines-Stroke is associated with sustained improvement in care for patients hospitalized with acute stroke or transient ischemic attack. Circulation. 2009; 119(1):107–115

[44] Lavados P. National Chilean Stroke Program. Presented at the I International Simposium of Stroke Neurology, Hospital de Clínicas de Porto Alegre. April 2017

[45] Sposato LA, Esnaola MM, Zamora R, Zurrú MC, Fustinoni O, Saposnik G, ReNACer Investigators, Argentinian Neurological

Society. Quality of ischemic stroke care in emerging countries: the Argentinian National Stroke Registry (ReNACer). Stroke. 2008; 39(11):3036–3041

[46] Estol CJ, Esnaola y Rojas MM. Stroke in Argentina. Int J Stroke. 2010; 5(1):35–39

[47] Góngora-Rivera F. Perspective on stroke in Mexico. Medicina Universitaria. 2015; 17(68):184–187

[48] Cantú-Brito C, Majersik JJ, Sánchez BN, et al. Door-to-door capture of incident and prevalent stroke cases in Durango, Mexico: the Brain Attack Surveillance in Durango Study. Stroke. 2011; 42(3):601–606

[49] Cantú-Brito C, Ruiz-Sandoval JL, Murillo-Bonilla LM, et al. PREMIER Investigators. Acute care and one-year outcome of Mexican patients with first-ever acute ischemic stroke: the PREMIER study. Rev Neurol. 2010; 51(11):641–649

[50] Ko KF, Sheppard L, Ko KF1. The contribution of a comprehensive stroke unit to the outcome of Chinese stroke patients. Singapore Med J. 2006; 47(3):208–212

[51] Wu B, Liu M, Liu H, et al. Meta-analysis of traditional Chinese patent medicine for ischemic stroke. Stroke. 2007; 38(6): 1973–9

[52] Mishra NK, Khadilkar SV. Stroke program for India. Ann Indian Acad Neurol. 2010; 13(1):28–32

[53] Pandian JD, Sudhan P. Stroke epidemiology and stroke care services in India. J Stroke. 2013; 15(3):128–134

[54] Cong NH. Stroke care in Vietnam. Int J Stroke. 2007; 2(4): 279–280

[55] Ringelstein EB, Chamorro A, Kaste M, et al. ESO Stroke Unit Certification Committee. European Stroke Organisation recommendations to establish a stroke unit and stroke center. Stroke. 2013; 44(3):828–840

[56] Krishnamurthi RV, Feigin VL, Forouzanfar MH, et al. Global Burden of Diseases, Injuries, Risk Factors Study 2010 (GBD 2010), GBD Stroke Experts Group. Global and regional burden of first-ever ischaemic and haemorrhagic stroke during 1990–2010: findings from the Global Burden of Disease Study 2010. Lancet Glob Health. 2013; 1(5):e259–e281

[57] Kunst AE, Amiri M, Janssen F. The decline in stroke mortality: exploration of future trends in 7 Western European countries. Stroke. 2011; 42(8):2126–2130

[58] Audebert HJ, Kukla C, Clarmann von Claranau S, et al. TEMPiS Group. Telemedicine for safe and extended use of thrombolysis in stroke: the Telemedic Pilot Project for Integrative Stroke Care (TEMPiS) in Bavaria. Stroke. 2005; 36(2):287–291

3 Emergency Stroke Care in the Prehospital Setting and Emergency Department

Charles M. Andrews, David French, and Dustin P. LeBlanc

Abstract

Most patients with stroke-like symptoms present to hospitals by prehospital care and emergency medical services (EMS). EMS plays a key role in the detection of stroke and further activation of the stroke system of care. Assessment of patients can be done with several prehospital scales aimed at rapid and correct evaluation. As endovascular stroke care becomes more available, EMS will also play a key role in transportation of stroke patients to specific facilities. Once a patient arrives in an Emergency Department, a prepared team will help move the patient through rapid imaging and further evaluation for potential IV thrombolysis and/or endovascular options. This must occur in an organized and protocolized format to ensure the most rapid care for all stroke patients.

Keywords: emergency medical services (EMS), prehospital stroke assessment, transport of stroke patients, stroke imaging, stroke systems of care, telemedicine, team-based care

3.1 Introduction

According to the 2018 American Heart Association/American Stroke Association (AHA/ASA) statistics, someone in the United States has a stroke roughly every 40 seconds, accounting for one of every 19 deaths annually and ranking fifth in leading causes of death. Although between 2005 and 2015, the age-adjusted stroke death rate decreased 21.7%, and the actual number of deaths declined by 2.3%, it remains a leading cause of serious long-term disability.[1] While advances have been made in the treatment of stroke, early recognition and presentation for diagnosis and treatment remain a challenge. Often this is accomplished through the activation of emergency medical services (EMS). While treatment upon arrival is often focused on the door-to-treatment time, EMS may improve the onset-to-door time through rapid assessment and stabilization of the patient and transport to an appropriate destination facility.

As the EMS system is frequently the entry point for stroke care, it plays a crucial role in the AHA chain of survival: Detection, Dispatch, Delivery, Door, Data, Decision, Drug, Disposition. From the early recognition of the signs of stroke, EMS must support critical hemodynamic processes (airway, breathing, circulation), make appropriate destination decisions, and alert the receiving facility with accurate and pertinent information to expedite treatment. Given the relatively narrow window of opportunity for treatment with systemic thrombolytics, EMS plays a crucial role in regional stroke systems.[2] In fact, there are many sources of delay in presentation of patients and thus ineligibility for acute reperfusion.[3] Factors associated with increased rates of reperfusion therapy include use of 911, EMS transport, severe symptoms, and first time stroke while decreased rates correlate to private transport, prior stroke history, mild symptoms, and rural locations.[4,5,6]

3.2 911 and EMS Dispatch

In order for patient management to begin, EMS must be activated by either the patient or a witness to the event. Through public education initiatives and outreach programs, the recognition of stroke symptoms is emphasized to include alterations in speech, weakness, or mentation.[2] Once these symptoms are recognized and 911 is activated, the initial point of contact is the emergency dispatcher or operator. Recognition of stroke as a potential diagnosis by the dispatcher is essential. While tools such as Emergency Medical Dispatch provide great assistance with recognition, there is still significant variability, with correct identification varying between 30 and 83%.[7] A well-organized regional stroke system not only educates dispatchers in recognition of stroke symptoms, but enables early notification of the receiving hospitals on impending arrivals, either through dispatch or EMS.

An AHA/ASA policy statement titled *Implementation Strategies for Emergency Medical Services Within Stroke Systems of Care* has identified the following parameters as measurements of quality from the EMS System (EMSS):

- Stroke patients are dispatched at the highest level of care available in the shortest time possible
- The time between the receipt of the call and the dispatch of the response team is < 90 seconds

- EMSS response time is < 8 minutes
- Dispatch time is < 1 minute
- Turnout time is < 1 minute
- The on-scene time is < 15 minutes
- Travel time is equivalent to trauma or acute myocardial infarction calls[2]

3.3 EMS Assessment

The initial primary survey of a stroke patient by EMS providers has the same priorities as other disease processes: Airway, Breathing, and Circulation. The presence of deficits in head and neck innervation may make secretion management more difficult and increase the risk of aspiration. Additionally, in ischemic strokes, higher blood pressures are tolerated, as they may be required to perfuse the penumbra. However, extreme hypertension (> 220 mm Hg systolic) may be treated in consultation with medical control. Respiratory depression is less common, but oxygenation and ventilation can be supported as necessary. Hyperventilation as a therapy should be avoided in the absence of signs of impending brain herniation given the risk of decreased cerebral perfusion. Special attention should be paid to circulatory status and ECG, given the association between cardiac arrhythmias and stroke. Additionally, blood glucose levels are routinely assessed, as hypoglycemia may mimic stroke-like symptoms. Intervention should include, if possible, an intravenous line amenable to the administration of medication as well as contrast material for diagnostic computer tomography (CT). However, none of these additional interventions should take priority over the rapid transport of the patient to an appropriate facility.[2]

History gathering may be difficult in a patient with aphasia or dysarthria, and supplemental history from family or witnesses should be gathered whenever possible. Critical history includes the "last known normal" or "last known well" time. This is the most recent point of time that the patient was without current stroke-like symptoms and represents "time zero" for the implementation of time-sensitive interventions such as thrombolytics. The "wake-up stroke" in which the patient awakens with symptoms presents an additional challenge, as the time used must correspond to when the patient was last known to be awake and symptom free, often prior to bed the night before. Additional points of history should include past medical history (e.g., prior stroke, seizure disorder, atrial fibrillation, or diabetes) as well as a medica-

tion history with special focus on systemic anticoagulants.[2] Concomitantly with these interventions and history points, a validated stroke screening and severity tool should be utilized.

3.4 Assessment Tools

For the detection of stroke symptoms by EMS, the patient should undergo an examination with a validated stroke assessment tool. These tools can be broken down into two broad categories: Screening and Severity tools. A wide variety of these tools exist, with the most common screening tools being the Cincinnati Prehospital Stroke Scale (CPSS) and Los Angeles Prehospital Stroke Scale (LAPSS). These tools include simple assessments for strength, facial droop, and speech, while the LAPSS includes limited historical factors. These tools are used in a binary fashion to detect positive stroke symptoms but were not designed to assess symptom severity. In a systematic review of these scales, it was found that the LAPSS was more consistent but had similar diagnostic capabilities to the CPSS. The accuracy of these tests varies, with up to 30% of strokes being missed.[3]

With the latest update of the AHA/ASA guidelines, there is an increased focus on recognition of large vessel occlusions (LVO), as these are more likely to be amenable to endovascular therapy.[8] Therefore, there has been an increased focused on the detection of LVO by the implementation of field-based stroke severity tools to ensure transport of these patients to facilities capable of performing endovascular interventions. These tools include the Cincinnati Stroke Triage Assessment Tool (CSTAT), Field Assessment Stroke Triage for Emergency Destination (FAST-ED), Los Angeles Motor Scale (LAMS) and Rapid Arterial Occlusion Evaluation (RACE) scale. These tools are based off the findings of the National Institutes of Health Stroke Scale (NIHSS), but are less detailed, more brief, and more suitable to the prehospital environment.[9] The specific test utilized in a given area depends on local preferences and protocols.

(▶ Table 3.1, ▶ Table 3.2, ▶ Table 3.3, ▶ Table 3.4)

3.5 Transport Destination

Once stroke symptoms have been detected and the severity assessed, the decision is made to transport the patient. The AHA/ASA guidelines designate three levels of hospitals based on their capabilities to provide care: Acute Stroke Ready Hospitals (ASRH), Primary Stroke Centers (PSC), and

Table 3.1 Cincinnati Prehospital Stroke Severity Scale

Conjugate gaze deviation	2 points
Incorrectly answers <u>Age</u> or <u>Month</u> **and** Does not follow at least one command (close your eyes, open and close your hand)	1 point
Arm (right, left or both) falls to the bed within 10 seconds	1 point

Score of **2 or more** = high likelihood of Large Vessel Occlusion (LVO) Stroke

Table 3.2 The FAST-ED scale and its corresponding NIHSS

Item	FAST-ED Score
Facial palsy	
Normal or minor paralysis	0
Partial or complete paralysis	1
Arm weakness	
No drift	0
Drift or some effort against gravity	1
No effort against gravity or no movement	2
Speech changes	
Absent	0
Mild to moderate	1
Severe, global aphasia, or mute	2
Gaze or eye deviation	
Absent	0
Partial	1
Forced deviation	2
Denial/Neglect	
Absent	0
Extinction to bilateral simultaneous stimulation in only one sensory modality	1
Does not recognize own hand or orients only to one side of the body	2

FAST-ED Indicates Field Assessment Stroke Triage Destination; and NIHSS, National Institutes of Health Stroke System

Comprehensive Stroke Centers (CSC). ASRHs are facilities previously referred to as "stroke-capable hospitals." This term is used for facilities that have made a commitment to effectively and efficiently evaluate, diagnose, and treat most emergency department (ED) stroke patients. These facilities may have treatment protocols, written transfer agreements with higher-level facilities, the ability to administer intravenous recombinant tissue plasminogen activator (rtPA), CT imaging, as well as integration into large stroke care systems via telemedicine or teleradiology. This has made possible the ability to increase service to rural areas by the "drip and ship" approach of evaluating patients with remote assistance from stroke specialists, administering rtPA, and then transferring to higher-level facilities for further care.

PSCs are facilities that have made a systematic commitment to stroke care and are required to closely track their performance metrics. These facilities statistically provide better care than their non-certified counterparts, with improved door to physician time, door to CT time, and door to intervention time. CSCs are facilities that are capable of offering state-of-the-art care at all times, with inclusion of neurocritical care units and additional specialty care. These facilities often exist as the center of a "hub and spoke" model of stroke care with outlying ASRHs or PSCs feeding into the CSC.[2]

Recently, the Joint Commission (JC) has recognized the increasing importance of access to endovascular therapy and developed a Thrombectomy-Capable Stroke Center (TSC) designation. This level of care falls between the PSC and CSC levels, focusing on mechanical thrombectomy and associated quality metrics.[10] Thrombectomy stroke centers or TSCs will aim to provide rapid procedural management (mechanical thrombectomy) but do not have the same capabilities as comprehensive centers making their impact unclear in the future. CSC have dedicated stroke units, neurocritical care and are centers of excellence that help nearby PSC and coordinate stroke care for example. TSCs that can perform a procedure but not deal with potential complications or complex cases provides potential benefit but without a known risk.

Geography often determines the ability of prehospital providers to transport a patient to varying levels of care. In the United States, 81% of the population has access by ground transport to a hospital capable of administering rtPA. Ground transport can access an endovascular-capable facility in the same time for 56%. By air, intravenous and endovascular capable centers are accessible to 97% and 85%, respectively, within one hour. Increasing the time range to 120 minutes, 99% of the population has access to both types of intervention. This transport time underlines the importance of acute symptom recognition by patients in order to reach destination facilities in a timely manner, and in some instances, use of helicopter EMS (HEMS) may be justified to deliver patients to a higher level of care in a timelier manner.

Given the often longer transport times to CSCs, consideration must be given to the likelihood of

Table 3.3 Comparison of Los Angeles Motor Score and NIH Stroke Score

LAMS	Score the affected side	Description	Corresponding NIHSS score
Facial Droop	0 Absent	No facial asymmetry. Normal.	Facial palsy 0–1
	1 Present	Partial or complete lower facial droop.	Facial palsy 2–3
Arm Drift	0 Absent	No drifts. Normal.	Motor arm 0 (normal)
	1 Drifts down	Drifts down but does not hit the bed within 10 seconds.	Motor arm 1 (drift)
	2 Falls rapidly	Arm cannot be held up against gravity and falls to the bed within 10 seconds.	Motor arm 2–4
Grip strength	0 Normal	Normal.	No NIHSS for this. Scored 0 if admission neuro exam rated grip strength as 5 (normal)
	1 weak grip	Weak but some movement.	Admission neuro exam rated grip strength as 4 (weak), 3 (some movement, but not against gravity)
	2 no grip	No movement. Muscle contraction be seen but without movement.	Neuro exam rated grip strength as 1 (muscle contraction but no movement) or 0 (no muscle contraction)
Total	= ___(Range 0–5)		A score ≥ 4 is highly predicted of large artery occlusion

benefit of intervention versus delay in arrival due to distance. Patients with higher severity scores are more likely to benefit from transport to a CSC.[11] Given this finding, the latest AHA/ASA transport recommendations state that patients with suspected LVO with last known normal time within 6 hours should proceed to a CSC if this will not increase transport time by more than 15 minutes. How TSCs are incorporated into this matrix remains to be seen. Regardless of mode of transport and destination facility, early notification by EMS is critical to timely intervention.[12]

3.6 Future

Stroke is an extremely time-sensitive disease process, and, as such, any time savings en route to diagnosis and treatment may confer significant advantages. Advances in technology have offered early access to further diagnostic tools. The prehospital use of *telestroke* with bidirectional audio-video communication to allow for evaluation of stroke patients while en route is becoming more widely available with improved mobile data networks. Additionally, diagnostic "mobile stroke units" have been implemented in several cities in the United States and abroad, with CT scanners on board special ambulances to provide rapid access

to diagnostic imaging and initiation of rtPA. Given the significant expense of these units, cost-effectiveness determinations regarding this approach are still lacking. Further diagnostic potential lies with the use of prehospital transcranial ultrasound. This method is noninvasive, nonradiating, and less expensive than CT scanning. However, several limitations currently exist to widespread implementation, including a lack of contrast agents in the United States, limited funding and access to equipment, validation of scanning protocols and training of practitioners in this technique.[13,14]

3.7 Emergency Department Management

More than 80% of acute stroke patients present to the ED, with very few presenting as inpatients.[15] Arrival to the ED can occur by variety of transportation methods, with EMS challenges aforementioned. Despite public education, a significant number of patients still arrive by private vehicle, which can delay triage, notification, and ultimately treatment.[16] The emergency physician's role is to provide rapid evaluation, diagnosis, and treatment and to offer guidance of hospital resources. Every aspect of ED care is essential and intended to allow for the best chance of timely therapy with tPA and

Table 3.4 RACE Scale

1. Facial palsy:	
Facial movement is normal, symmetric	0
Facial gesture when showing the teeth or smiling is slightly asymmetrical	1
Facial gesture when showing the teeth or smiling is completely asymmetrical	2
2. Arm motor function:	
Can maintain the arm against gravity > 10 seconds	0
Can maintain the arm against gravity < 10 seconds	1
Cannot maintain the leg against gravity and drops immediately	2
3. Leg motor function:	
Can maintain the leg against gravity > 5 seconds	0
Can maintain the leg against gravity < 5 seconds	1
Cannot maintain the leg against gravity and drops immediately	2
4. Head and gaze deviation	
Absent	0
Present	1
5.A. Agnosia/Negligence	
Asomatognosia (does not recognize the left part of his/her body if left hemiparesis present). Anosognosia (does not recognize his/her weakness)	
No asomatognosia or anosognosia is present	0
Asomatognosia or anosognosia is present	1
There is no asomatognosia and anosognosia (both present)	2
5B. Aphasia/Language (if right hemiparesis)	
Ask the patient "Close your eyes" and "Make a fist"	
Perform both tasks correctly	0
Perform one task correctly	1
Perform neither task	2
TOTAL:	

thrombectomy. For this to occur, the system must be organized, streamlined and have invested individuals who care about the outcomes of stroke patients.

3.7.1 Team-Based Care

Emergency management of acute stroke is centered around a team-based approach with shared responsibilities and actions. Care teams often include members from emergency medicine, stroke neurology, pharmacy, radiology, nursing, laboratory services, and even admissions. Every individual's job on this team is crucial, but the emergency physician must provide leadership and shepherd the patient through the whole process. ▶ Fig. 3.1 demonstrates key steps along the process in the work-up of a patient with stroke-like symptoms.

Excellence in a stroke center requires more than implementation of a stroke team. These teams must track their metrics, receive feedback regularly on cases and address local barriers to care[17,18] to allow continual assessment and improvement. Most hospitals employ stroke protocols to ensure standards are met and that emergency staff are educated. Regional stroke services must also provide care to stroke patients from urban and rural populations alike. Often, stroke physicians are not immediately available in rural areas, and the emergency physician must be capable and comfortable with the diagnosis and treatment of stroke. As mentioned, advances in technology allow telemedicine services to provide much greater coverage to these areas as well as treatment.[19] Stroke care will always be team-based and require stroke champions within multiple disciplines of the hospital.

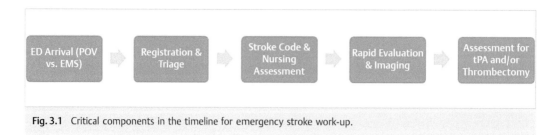

Fig. 3.1 Critical components in the timeline for emergency stroke work-up.

3.8 Systems of Care

Regionalization of stroke care has been accomplished in the last decade largely with the evidence supporting mechanical thrombectomy. This model is based on preexisting systems of care and greatly follows the regionalization of trauma care systems.[20] This model ensures not just a localized proximity to stroke care and specialists in a timely manner, but also a hierarchy for the severity of stroke. In the early 2000s it was clear that a majority of stroke patients presented outside of the tissue plasminogen activator (tPA) time window,[21] and very few of the public had any awareness regarding acute stroke symptoms or treatment options.[22] However, despite aggressive educational programs, presentation outside of the tPA time window still remains the most common reason to be ineligible for tPA.[23] Given recent trials demonstrating the benefit to mechanical thrombectomy not just within 6 hours[24,25,26,27,28,29] but also up to 24 hours,[30,31] more patients may be eligible for treatment. This has provoked the addition of thrombectomy-capable stroke centers distinct from primary and comprehensive stroke centers. Thus, access to these centers in a timely manner is critical to management. Many regionalized stroke networks have started to employ the use of telemedicine to allow expanded access. Prior to more widespread telemedicine usage, it was discovered that many small and rural hospitals in the South and Midwest had used tPA sparingly if at all.[32] In South Carolina, it was estimated that telemedicine increased the access to stroke experts within 60 minutes from 38% to 76%[19] and significantly improved stroke access throughout the state.

3.9 Stroke Imaging

All patients with suspected stroke-like symptoms must receive emergent brain imaging to differentiate hemorrhagic stroke from ischemic stroke. In a majority of institutions this will likely be CT imaging, given the availability and cost-effectiveness of MRI.[33,34] It is recommended by the AHA/ASA Stroke Guidelines that the goal for brain imaging should be less than 20 minutes.[35] This is based on the mantra that "time is brain" and that every minute without intervention, millions of neurons are lost.[36] Significant decreases in door-to-groin puncture times were found by "streamlining" stroke patients with interventions including feedback, direct communication lines, EMS prenotification, and direct transport to CT.[37] Several studies have found that processes that reduced door-to-CT are associated with increased use of tPA, reduced time to endovascular therapy, and improved outcomes.[38,39] Further specifics of stroke imaging will be covered in a later chapter of this book.

3.10 Emergency Management

Evaluation of the stroke patient in the ED is first focused on the ABCs and similar to any other patient. Patients must have an assessment of their airway, breathing, and circulation, in rapid succession. Given the trend towards door-to-CT imaging, the emergency physician must often evaluate the patient in CT or en route to ensure clinical stability. If the patient is obtunded and not protecting the airway, a decision must be made to allow rapid CT imaging followed by intubation and mechanical ventilation or to secure the airway first. Patients who must be have their airway secured may have delays in CT imaging and ultimately reperfusion, thus the delay must be warranted. Blood glucose is the only required lab prior to consideration of thrombolysis.[35] Other diagnostic labs including coagulation studies, and platelets may necessary given clinical suspicion or history. Physicians must recognize alterations in blood pressure and work to quickly correct them. Hypotension may be present when ischemic strokes are secondary to underlying diagnoses such as sepsis, myocardial infarctions, heart failure, and hypovolemia. Small nonrandomized trials have looked at vasopressors in ischemic stroke and found that they improve perfusion, but none have shown clinical or outcome benefit.[40] One must also understand that there exists a U-shaped relationship with blood pressure in stroke and that high as well as low pressures are associated with death and dependency.[41] Current stroke guidelines recommend lowering systolic blood pressure to ≤ 185 and diastolic to ≤ 110 mm Hg, prior to any thrombolysis.[35] Optimal agents for rapid reduction to goal blood pressures include drugs such as labetalol and nicardipine, but any drug with rapid onset of action and easy titration is favorable. Stroke guidelines also recommend the use of NIHSS for severity scoring.[35] In a patient who is eligible for tPA, and/or thrombectomy, rapid evaluation, which may not include the entire NIHSS, can be justified. For instance, a patient who is globally aphasic with right hemiplegia and a forced gaze preference very likely has a left middle cerebral artery occlusion and requires tPA and thrombectomy, while testing noncortical findings (ataxia, sensory, etc.) may lead to delays in treatment. This was the primary reason for the development of prehospital stroke scales, given their ease of use and speed in testing. Many stroke patients are found down or unresponsive, and physicians may consider cervical spine immobilization or cervical collars until clinical clearance can be obtained. Once a patient has been deemed eligible for thrombolysis, the emergency physician must be knowledgeable of the contraindications and capable of delivery of tPA without delay.

3.11 Conclusions

Emergency Departments and physicians are key in the delivery of excellent stroke care. EMS is the most common form of arrival for stroke patients, and rapid assessment, prenotification and delivery to appropriate stroke centers dramatically influences treatment times. Telemedicine is becoming more commonly used both prehospital and in the ED to improve access to stroke physicians. The emergency physician must be capable of delivering timely stroke care and assisting in treatment.

References

[1] Benjamin EJ, Virani SS, Callaway CW, et al. American Heart Association Council on Epidemiology and Prevention Statistics Committee and Stroke Statistics Subcommittee. Heart Disease and Stroke Statistics-2018 Update: A Report From the American Heart Association. Circulation. 2018; 137(12): e67–e492

[2] Jauch EC, Saver JL, Adams HP, Jr, et al. American Heart Association Stroke Council, Council on Cardiovascular Nursing, Council on Peripheral Vascular Disease, Council on Clinical Cardiology. Guidelines for the early management of patients with acute ischemic stroke: a guideline for healthcare professionals from the American Heart Association/American Stroke Association. Stroke. 2013; 44(3):870–947

[3] Fassbender K, Balucani C, Walter S, Levine SR, Haass A, Grotta J. Streamlining of prehospital stroke management: the golden hour. Lancet Neurol. 2013; 12(6):585–596

[4] Higashida R, Alberts MJ, Alexander DN, et al. American Heart Association Advocacy Coordinating Committee. Interactions within stroke systems of care: a policy statement from the American Heart Association/American Stroke Association. Stroke. 2013; 44(10):2961–2984

[5] Gebhardt JG, Norris TE. Acute stroke care at rural hospitals in Idaho: challenges in expediting stroke care. J Rural Health. 2006; 22(1):88–91

[6] Mullen MT, Wiebe DJ, Bowman A, et al. Disparities in accessibility of certified primary stroke centers. Stroke. 2014; 45 (11):3381–3388

[7] Kimball MM, Neal D, Waters MF, Hoh BL. Race and income disparity in ischemic stroke care: nationwide inpatient sample database, 2002 to 2008. J Stroke Cerebrovasc Dis. 2014; 23(1):17–24

[8] Brandler ES, Sharma M, Sinert RH, Levine SR. Prehospital stroke scales in urban environments: a systematic review. Neurology. 2014; 82(24):2241–2249

[9] Powers WJ, Derdeyn CP, Biller J, et al. American Heart Association Stroke Council. 2015 American Heart Association/American Stroke Association Focused Update of the 2013 Guidelines for the Early Management of Patients With Acute Ischemic Stroke Regarding Endovascular Treatment: A Guideline for Healthcare Professionals From the American Heart Association/American Stroke Association. Stroke. 2015; 46 (10):3020–3035

[10] Krebs W, Sharkey-Toppen TP, Cheek F, et al. Prehospital Stroke Assessment for Large Vessel Occlusions: A Systematic Review. Prehosp Emerg Care. 2018; 22(2):180–188

[11] Adeoye O, Albright KC, Carr BG, et al. Geographic access to acute stroke care in the United States. Stroke. 2014; 45(10): 3019–3024

[12] Schlemm E, Ebinger M, Nolte CH, Endres M, Schlemm L. Optimal Transport Destination for Ischemic Stroke Patients With Unknown Vessel Status: Use of Prehospital Triage Scores. Stroke. 2017; 48(8):2184–2191

[13] Crocco TJ. Streamlining stroke care: from symptom onset to emergency department. J Emerg Med. 2007; 33(3):255–260

[14] Yperzeele L, Van Hooff RJ, De Smedt A, et al. Prehospital stroke care: limitations of current interventions and focus on new developments. Cerebrovasc Dis. 2014; 38(1):1–9

[15] Cumbler E. In-Hospital Ischemic Stroke. Neurohospitalist. 2015; 5(3):173–181

[16] Mohammad YM. Mode of arrival to the emergency department of stroke patients in the United States. J Vasc Interv Neurol. 2008; 1(3):83–86

[17] Dirks M, Niessen LW, van Wijngaarden JD, et al. PRomoting ACute Thrombolysis in Ischemic StrokE (PRACTISE) Investigators. Promoting thrombolysis in acute ischemic stroke. Stroke. 2011; 42(5):1325–1330

[18] Scott PA, Meurer WJ, Frederiksen SM, et al. INSTINCT Investigators. A multilevel intervention to increase community hospital use of alteplase for acute stroke (INSTINCT): a

cluster-randomised controlled trial. Lancet Neurol. 2013; 12 (2):139–148

[19] Magarik JA, Jauch EC, Patel SJ, et al. MUSC's comprehensive stroke program: changing what's possible in stroke care across South Carolina. J S C Med Assoc. 2012; 108(5):128–131

[20] Fargen KM, Jauch E, Khatri P, et al. Needed dialog: regionalization of stroke systems of care along the trauma model. Stroke. 2015; 46(6):1719–1726

[21] Kleindorfer D, de los Rios La Rosa F, Khatri P, Kissela B, Mackey J, Adeoye O. Temporal trends in acute stroke management. Stroke. 2013; 44(6) Suppl 1:S129–S131

[22] Kleindorfer D, Khoury J, Broderick JP, et al. Temporal trends in public awareness of stroke: warning signs, risk factors, and treatment. Stroke. 2009; 40(7):2502–2506

[23] Barber PA, Zhang J, Demchuk AM, Hill MD, Buchan AM. Why are stroke patients excluded from TPA therapy? An analysis of patient eligibility. Neurology. 2001; 56(8):1015–1020

[24] Berkhemer OA, Fransen PS, Beumer D, et al. MR CLEAN Investigators. A randomized trial of intraarterial treatment for acute ischemic stroke. N Engl J Med. 2015; 372(1):11–20

[25] Goyal M, Demchuk AM, Menon BK, et al. ESCAPE Trial Investigators. Randomized assessment of rapid endovascular treatment of ischemic stroke. N Engl J Med. 2015; 372(11):1019–1030

[26] Campbell BC, Mitchell PJ, Kleinig TJ, et al. EXTEND-IA Investigators. Endovascular therapy for ischemic stroke with perfusion-imaging selection. N Engl J Med. 2015; 372(11):1009–1018

[27] Jovin TG, Chamorro A, Cobo E, et al. REVASCAT Trial Investigators. Thrombectomy within 8 hours after symptom onset in ischemic stroke. N Engl J Med. 2015; 372(24):2296–2306

[28] Saver JL, Goyal M, Bonafe A, et al. SWIFT PRIME Investigators. Stent-retriever thrombectomy after intravenous t-PA vs. t-PA alone in stroke. N Engl J Med. 2015; 372(24):2285–2295

[29] Bracard S, Ducrocq X, Mas JL, et al. THRACE investigators. Mechanical thrombectomy after intravenous alteplase versus alteplase alone after stroke (THRACE): a randomised controlled trial. Lancet Neurol. 2016; 15(11):1138–1147

[30] Albers GW, Marks MP, Kemp S, et al. DEFUSE 3 Investigators. Thrombectomy for Stroke at 6 to 16 Hours with Selection by Perfusion Imaging. N Engl J Med. 2018; 378(8):708–718

[31] Nogueira RG, Jadhav AP, Haussen DC, et al. DAWN Trial Investigators. Thrombectomy 6 to 24 Hours after Stroke with a Mismatch between Deficit and Infarct. N Engl J Med. 2018; 378(1):11–21

[32] Kleindorfer D, Xu Y, Moomaw CJ, Khatri P, Adeoye O, Hornung R. US geographic distribution of rt-PA utilization by hospital for acute ischemic stroke. Stroke. 2009; 40(11): 3580–3584

[33] Brazzelli M, Sandercock PA, Chappell FM, et al. Magnetic resonance imaging versus computed tomography for detection of acute vascular lesions in patients presenting with stroke symptoms. Cochrane Database Syst Rev. 2009 (4):CD007424

[34] Wardlaw J, Brazzelli M, Miranda H, et al. An assessment of the cost-effectiveness of magnetic resonance, including diffusion-weighted imaging, in patients with transient ischaemic attack and minor stroke: a systematic review, meta-analysis and economic evaluation. Health Technol Assess. 2014; 18 (27):1–368, v–vi.

[35] Powers WJ, Rabinstein AA, Ackerson T, et al. American Heart Association Stroke Council. 2018 Guidelines for the Early Management of Patients With Acute Ischemic Stroke: A Guideline for Healthcare Professionals From the American Heart Association/American Stroke Association. Stroke. 2018; 49 (3):e46–e110

[36] Saver JL. Time is brain–quantified. Stroke. 2006; 37(1):263–266

[37] Aghaebrahim A, Streib C, Rangaraju S, et al. Streamlining door to recanalization processes in endovascular stroke therapy. J Neurointerv Surg. 2017; 9(4):340–345

[38] Messé SR, Khatri P, Reeves MJ, et al. Why are acute ischemic stroke patients not receiving IV tPA? Results from a national registry. Neurology. 2016; 87(15):1565–1574

[39] Saver JL, Goyal M, van der Lugt A, et al. HERMES Collaborators. Time to Treatment With Endovascular Thrombectomy and Outcomes From Ischemic Stroke: A Meta-analysis. JAMA. 2016; 316(12):1279–1288

[40] Mistri AK, Robinson TG, Potter JF. Pressor therapy in acute ischemic stroke: systematic review. Stroke. 2006; 37(6): 1565–1571

[41] Leonardi-Bee J, Bath PM, Phillips SJ, Sandercock PA, Group ISTC, IST Collaborative Group. Blood pressure and clinical outcomes in the International Stroke Trial. Stroke. 2002; 33 (5):1315–1320

4 Imaging Techniques in Acute Ischemic Stroke

Nicolás Sgarbi

Abstract

Acute ischemic stroke is a real health problem with a significant morbidity and mortality. In the last years there were importat modifications in therapeutic results with positive impact in patients outcome. To obtain the appropiate results it is of great importance to make a detail patient selection. This selection lies on a lot of clinical and imaging information in the hypercaute phase. Neuroimaging with CT and/or MRI plays a key role in the study of a patient with ischemic stroke in the first hours of evolution with emphasis on patient selection to different therapeutics modalities.

Keywords: acute ischemic stroke imaing, computed tomography, magnetic resonance imaging, difusion, perfusion

4.1 Introduction

Acute ischemic stroke (AIS) is at present a high-ranking health problem on account of the high percentage of the population it affects and the sequels it can determine.

During the last few years the approach to this disease has undergone considerable modification, mainly on account of the publication of numerous clinical trials[1,2] demonstrating excellent therapeutic results.

Clearly, the main therapeutic objectives are to restore blood flow in the affected area and to decrease the effect of ischemia on tissue.[3]

The main change has taken place at the hyperacute stage, where the introduction of different protocols of patient selection and their corresponding treatment guidelines have had an impact on the prognosis regarding survival and functional abilities.[4]

While therapy progressed, different imaging techniques provided substantial information as a basis for therapeutic protocols and also for a better understanding of this pathology.[5]

Imaging has opened up, consequently, a series of possibilities: accurate diagnosis of ischemia or ischemia-like diseases (differential diagnoses), identification of potentially salvageable tissue (penumbra or tissue at risk for ischemia), localization of vascular occlusion and analysis of same, and finally selection of patients to be treated during the hyperacute phase and choice of the corresponding imaging method.[1]

AIS is, beyond doubt, a medical emergency. Therefore, the chosen imaging method must be quickly and accurately performed and promptly interpreted, so as not to delay treatment.

A subject of extensive discussion in the last few years is which would be the best method and how to select patients for it.

Regarding the first stages, the choice between computed tomography (CT) and magnetic resonance (MR) has been the subject of much discussion and analysis.[6] It has been clearly demonstrated that CT is excellent at detecting hemorrhage while MR is the most sensitive detector of ischemia at the hyperacute stage.[7]

As we shall see later on, MR is beyond doubt the most complete method for the study of AIS patients at the hyperacute stage, but its use in an emergency setting poses such logistic problems that many centers keep it as a resource for specific situations.[7] Notwithstanding, the last years have seen a trend toward the increasingly frequent use of MR as a basis for the choice of therapy, on account of its unique contributions.

We will review the present state of the different available imaging techniques for the study of AIS patients at the hyperacute stage and the impact of those techniques on choice and therapeutic management of patients.

4.2 Objectives of Imaging Methods

Neuroimaging plays an important role in the study of a stroke patient and affects therapy in a significant way. That is why most of the algorithms proposed in clinical trials include criteria or information derived from imaging.

The main objective of imaging methods, CT above all, is to establish a diagnosis of AIS in a patient and discard possible differential diagnoses or mimics. Notwithstanding, in the last few years different therapeutic options have provided evidence that has considerably modified the objectives of imaging.

The assessment of parenchyma, the absence of hemorrhage (main contraindication of the use of fibrinolytics) and the confirmation of ischemia are all important, but they are not the only factors. It is also essential to assess the state of brain circulation regarding the vascular tree itself and the main hemodynamic parameters.[8]

There is no consensus on the imaging method of choice for the selection of AIS patients. In spite of that, it is clear that the chosen method must provide information quickly in order to screen patients adequately for early treatment.

The AHA recommends both CT and MR as methods of choice in patients clinically suspected for hyperacute ischemia. Therefore they should be considered as methods providing complementary information. A guideline should not determine which method is the most adequate one.

After ruling out hemorrhage, it is basic to define whether confirmed ischemia is present and its extension, that is to say the size of the infarct core. As we will see later on, this is a key parameter for the first therapeutic decisions.

Another basic point is the detection of occlusion in a main cerebral artery (a proximal occlusion). The best parameters for patient prognosis are precisely the detection of occlusion and the neurological findings.[9]

At the present moment it is also necessary to evaluate potentially recoverable tissue, what is called the penumbra area, which is the main target of reperfusion therapies.

Although PET has been established as the gold standard for the definition of ischemic area and penumbra area, it cannot enter daily clinical practice. That is why we have reviewed the contribution of both CT and multimodal MR to the definition and evaluation of those parameters.

4.3 Analysis of Brain Parenchyma: Infarct Core

When a patient presents with a probable AIS at the hyperacute stage the first and basic step is to ascertain the state of the cerebral parenchyma.

Once hemorrhage has been excluded, the existence or absence of ischemia must be ascertained quickly; if ischemia is present, its extension must be defined, because it will constitute the infarct core.

The presence and extension of irreversibly damaged tissue is one of the factors that determines prognosis.

Non-contrast CT is clearly established as the method of first choice and must be performed

immediately in AIS is suspected (Class I, Level of Evidence A).[10] The main objectives remain the elimination of differential diagnoses and mimics of brain ischemia, and the exclusion of hemorrhage, which is the main contraindication for revascularization treatments.

Contrast CT is highly sensitive for the diagnosis of parenchymal and subarachnoid hemorrhage. It is therefore sufficient to exclude patients with these pathologies from reperfusion treatments.[1]

Non-contrast CT has long been accepted as being sufficient in itself as the single method to decide the use of intravenous thrombolytics in AIS patients (Class I, Level of evidence A).[11,12]

Although this is a firmly established principle, CT is a low-performance procedure for the diagnosis of ischemia in the first hours after its onset. CT performance depends likewise from the location of the infarcted areas.[13,14]

Within the first 3 to 6 hours of established ischemia, which is the critical period for the selection of patients, CT signs are very subtle; the scan is usually normal.

As the hours go by, ischemic areas show up on CT. Some 36–48 hours after the clinical onset, the compromised areas are visible as well-defined hypodense zones in 100% of cases.[15]

At the hyperacute stage it is of the essence to be able to detect the so-called early ischemic signs on CT. These signs must be quantified.

Early ischemia signs include: effacement of lentiform nucleus, loss of gray-white differentiation at the insula (insular ribbon sign), localized loss of differentiation between white and gray matter and localized effacement of sulci. (► Fig. 4.1)

Another high-ranking sign is hyperdensity of the middle cerebral artery. This sign does not indicate the presence of ischemia, but it locates the vascular occlusion responsible for the affected area and usually correlates with a proximal thrombus (at the M1 segment of the above mentioned artery). (► Fig. 4.2)

Although this sign has been described for other arteries in the cerebral circulation, it does not perform or correlate so well in those cases.

It is important to remember that this is a low-sensitivity sign and that false positives do appear, in patients with high hematocrit or in cases with severe atheromatosis with calcified vessel walls, for example.

It has been pointed out that undoubtedly the perception of early AIS signs is highly variable, from one observer to another and even for the same observer.

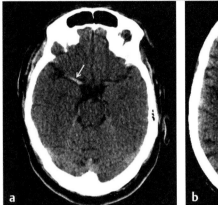
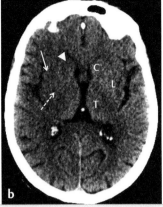
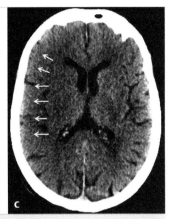

Fig. 4.1 Early ischemic signs in non-contrast CT. (a) Hyperdense middle cerebral artery sign (arrow) in evidence on the right side. The patient had presented with left motor impairment of 60 minutes' duration. **(b)** Early signs include: effacement of the caput of the right caudate nucleus (arrowhead), loss of the white-gray differentiation at the insula or insular ribbon sign (arrow) and effacement of the lenticular nucleus (dotted arrow). **(c)** Caput of caudate nucleus/L: lenticular nucleus/T: thalamus **(c)** Note the effacement or loss of white-gray differentiation on the superficial territory of the right middle cerebral artery (arrows).

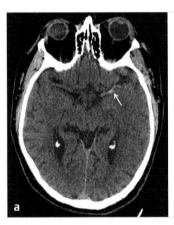
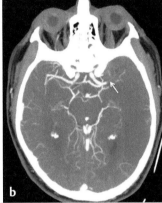

Fig. 4.2 Hyperdense middle cerebral artery sign. The sign is in evidence in **(a)**, indicating the presence of a thrombus in the proximal segment of the right middle cerebral artery (arrow) and its counterpart in the angio-CT scan, **(b)** A filling defect on the same spot. This makes it possible to diagnose a proximal occlusion promptly and then to develop the best therapeutic strategy.

Global sensitivity for these signs during the early period (3 hours) amounts to 30–60%, specificity being around 85%; the negative predictive value is very low, less than 30%.

When the area is clearly identifiable as ischemic, it will present to the eye of the observer as a hypodense zone with loss of gray-white differentiation and a well-defined margin. It is also clearly part of an arterial vascular territory.

Strategies have been devised to quantify the areas of ischemic tissue, which would be a means of patient selection. The ASPECTS (Alberta Stroke Program Early CT score) score is one of them; it allows the quantification of irreversibly damaged tissue in a simple way for patients with middle cerebral artery compromise.[16]

The use of ASPECTS for the selection of patients soon prevailed. Although the extension of ischemic areas does not exclude the patient from treatment, it does exert a significant influence on prognosis. Consequently, low-score patients with the corresponding zones of confirmed ischemia are excluded from early reperfusion therapy.

It has been demonstrated that the use of ASPECTS has some limitations, mainly regarding the borders of affected zones and the concept of volume (singly considered) correlating poorly with prognosis.

Notwithstanding, the ASPECTS concept is widely used at present, even if MR is the preferred method.

MR is a method of high sensitivity and specificity for the diagnosis of ischemia in the early hours

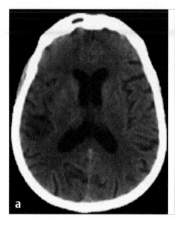 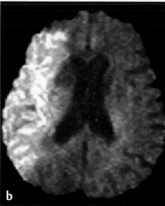

Fig. 4.3 Diffusion techniques, CT versus MR. MR, particularly if combined with DWI and ADC mapping, is the technique of choice for the diagnosis of early ischemia. This study corresponds to a patient with left motor impairment of 45 minutes' duration. **(a)** The non-contrast CT scan shows no alterations. **(b)** The DWI sequence is positive for cytotoxic edema in the whole right middle cerebral artery territory.

after onset, especially since the introduction of diffusion–weighted imaging and apparent diffusion coefficient mapping (DWI/ADC).[9,17]

On this ground among others, many centers have decided to use MR as a method for the selection of patients.

The DWI/ADC sequence can evaluate the movements of water molecules, which are limited or restricted on account of neuronal membrane alterations produced by brain ischemia.[17]

The sensitivity and specificity of the DWI/ADC sequence for the detection of ischemia in the first 6 hours is over 95% (Level of Evidence A). This diagnostic yield bears no relation to the volume or the location of the infarct. (▶ Fig. 4.3, ▶ Fig. 4.4)

According to available evidence this imaging modality can detect ischemia in less than 15 minutes after onset.

In clinical practice the tissue areas with restricted diffusion are considered unrecoverable. In spite of that, there have been reports of reversion of altered signals in such areas after reperfusion therapy.

Classically CT was spoken of as a method superior to MR for the detection of early-stage hemorrhage. Nevertheless, MR is similar in sensitivity and specificity to CT in the diagnosis of acute cerebral hemorrhage (Level of Evidence B).

In order to optimize diagnostic yield in this aspect it is basic to add susceptibility sequences (GRE T2 or SWI/SWAN) to the study protocol. These sequences also play a key role in the detection of asymptomatic micro-bleeds.[18]

These focal findings, which were considered of fundamental importance a few years ago, are now viewed differently: the presence of less than 5 micro-bleeds does not significantly increase the risk of symptomatic bleeding in patients treated with thrombolytics (Class IIa, Level of evidence B).

As mentioned above, once the ischemic areas have been identified, their extension must be quantified. (▶ Fig. 4.5)

Volume quantification of core or infarct nucleus (non-salvageable tissue) is of crucial prognostic importance: it is one of the highest-ranking independent predictive signs.

At present, it is firmly established that core volume, quantified by means of DWI/ADC, is one of the most influential factors for patient prognosis.[19]

A volume of 70–100 ml of ischemia in the territory of the middle cerebral artery is highly specific for poor outcome, independently from the existence of penumbra (potentially salvageable tissue) or a successful vascular recanalization.[20,21]

Furthermore, the risk of significant hemorrhage during treatment increases in proportion to the size of infarcted tissue, especially if the area is bigger than 100 ml.[22] That is why many authors do not recommend reperfusion therapy in this type of patient.

In spite of that fact, no precise cutoff point has been established that would enable to determine which patients should be excluded from reperfusion therapy, because there have been reports on favorable outcome for considerable ischemic areas after treatment.

4.4 Analysis of the Vascular Tree: Occlusion Level and Collateral Network

In a patient with hyperacute AIS, it is essential to study the status of the intracranial vascular tree. It

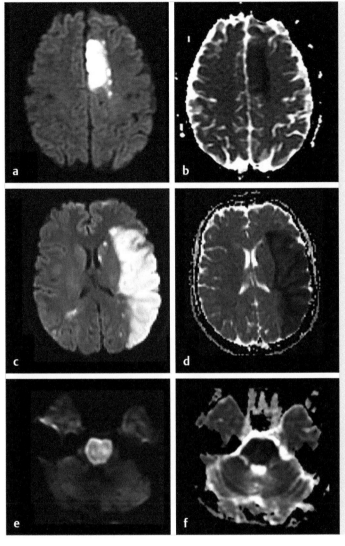

Fig. 4.4 DWI/ADC for the diagnosis of the ischemia core. The DWI sequence is the most sensitive technique for the assessment of the size and other features of the ischemic area, regardless of localization. **(a, b)** Show a superficial ischemic zone in the territory of the anterior cerebral artery; in **(c, d)** a completely ischemic area is noted in the territory of the left middle cerebral artery; and **(e, f)** show an infarct of the brain stem at pons level.

has been clearly established that this parameter impacts the taking of decisions in such patients.[23]

Detecting a proximal arterial occlusion is the primary objective of the non-invasive studies. Such techniques are recommended by the AHA (Class I, Level of Evidence A) before arterial endovascular treatment.[24]

The diagnostic contribution of both angiographic techniques, CTA and MRA, has been analyzed. The first study for most patients is non-contrast-enhanced CT, but CTA is very efficient for the retrieval of decisive information.

Both are recommended by the AHA (Class I, Level of Evidence A). (▶ Fig. 4.6)

Fast and easy acquisition makes CTA the favorite method in numerous centers, although MRA with

TOF technique is a highly sensitive and specific method for the detection of proximal occlusions.

CTA uses both iodinated contrast medium and radiations for data retrieval, two factors that have been unfavorably viewed. Notwithstanding, on account of its wide availability and easy performance it has become the modality of choice. The study usually starts at the aortic arch and goes up to the whole of the circle of Willis and its branches. 3D reconstructions on every spatial plane can be done with a high degree of anatomic resolution.

Detection of stenosis of varying degree can be accomplished at a high level of sensitivity and specificity, which has elevated CTA to the position of an indispensable technique for AIS patients.[25]

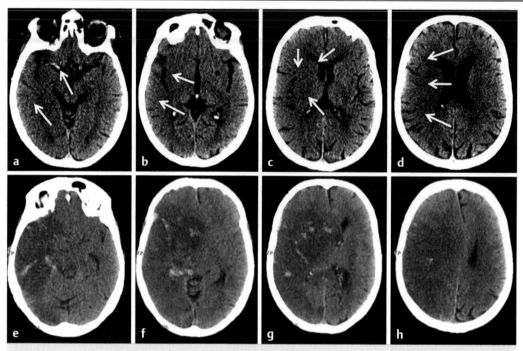

Fig. 4.5 Quantification of the ischemic area in the non-contrast CT scan. 62-year old patient presenting with sudden left hemiplegia 90 minutes ago. **(a-d)** Early ischemia signs in the non-contrast CT scan, with hyperdense middle cerebral artery sign on the right and an ASPECTS score of less than 7. Treatment with intravenous fibrinolytics was performed. Eight hours later the patient's level of consciousness decreases and he sinks into a coma. **(e-h)** Show the next CT evidencing hemorrhagic transformation and the malignant behavior of the ischemic area.

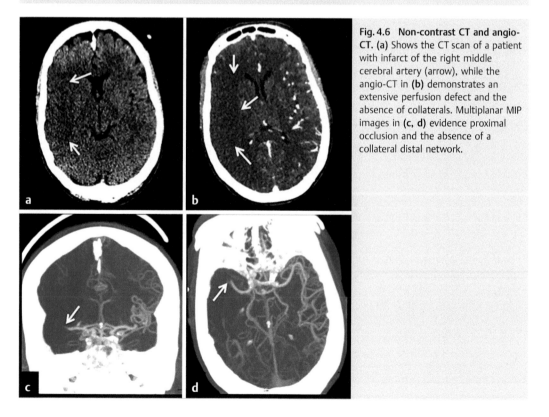

Fig. 4.6 Non-contrast CT and angio-CT. (a) Shows the CT scan of a patient with infarct of the right middle cerebral artery (arrow), while the angio-CT in **(b)** demonstrates an extensive perfusion defect and the absence of collaterals. Multiplanar MIP images in **(c, d)** evidence proximal occlusion and the absence of a collateral distal network.

CTA achieves, in fact, sensitivity and specificity over 95% as compared to digital subtraction angiography.[10,12,26]

Some centers prefer MRA as imaging modality because it does not use contrast medium and its overall performance is adequate for evaluation of occlusion level. Regarding the detection of proximal occlusions, sensitivity amounts to 84–87%, while specificity varies between 85% and 98%.[7,26]

Main limitations of this method are: significantly longer acquisition times and overestimation of stenosis, both linked to technical factors inherent to this modality.[26]

Another way of evaluating the level of occlusion is the susceptibility-weighted MR technique, such as the SWI/SWAN sequences.

Acute proximal thrombus is easily detected in these sequences, just as in non-contrast-enhanced CT, by means of the hyperdense artery sign ("susceptibility vessel sign").

The chosen angiographic method contributes another type of information: the analysis of collateral circulation.

It is quite clear that once a vascular occlusion is established, the size of the infarcted zone will depend not only on the level of the occlusion but also on the collateral network distal to it. Evaluation of the leptomeningeal network around the infarct core is beyond doubt important, because this network determines the presence or absence of penumbra areas and their size.

The so-called multiphase CTA permits a fast and easy visualization of the distal branches of the vascular tree and the collateral vessels acting as the patient's vascular reserve. (▶ Fig. 4.7)

It is a confirmed fact that good pial collaterals distal to a proximal occlusion correlate to a smaller infarct core and more potentially salvageable tissue, and consequently to a better outcome.

Different scoring systems for collateral network have been devised, based on CTA findings; their contribution has modified the evaluation of the intracranial vascular tree in AIS patients.

On this particular subject MRA is unimportant because of its low yield in the evaluation of the state of circulation distal to the circle of Willis, which adds another limiting feature to this modality.

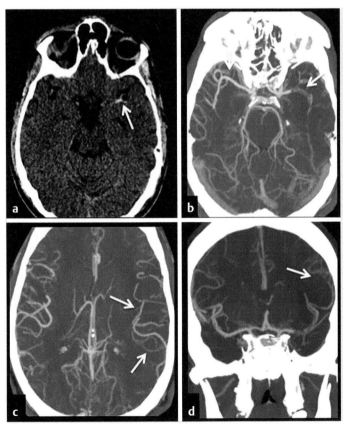

Fig. 4.7 Non-contrast CT and angio-CT. Patient whose right motor impairment began 45 minutes ago. **(a)** Non-contrast CT shows a hyperdense left middle cerebral artery (arrow). **(b-d)** MIP images of the angio-CT evidence proximal occlusion **(b**, arrow), while an excellent quantity of collaterals distal to the occlusion is demonstrated in **(c, d)** (arrow).

To resume, network status is an important prognostic factor, on the same level as initial NIHSS score and core size.

Collateral network status correlates to perfusion parameters, because the lower the level of brain blood volume, the lesser the operating network.

Bearing in mind these concepts it becomes clear that quality and quantity of leptomeningeal network correlates to core size and extension of potentially recoverable tissue, and on that account must be taken as a predictive factor for the patient's outcome.

4.5 Hemodynamic Analysis (Cerebral Perfusion): Penumbra Area

In the last few years the algorithms for the study and treatment of the AIS patient have undergone considerable change. These strategies include the implementation of Stroke Units and the use of revascularization therapy, both of which have had a positive impact in the management of the AIS patient at the hyperacute stage.

Two conditions are necessary for a better outcome: early recruitment of patients and identification and quantification of at-risk brain tissue (penumbra or potentially salvageable tissue).

The imaging approach has changed as well. Nowadays perfusion techniques play a major role in the paradigm of study and treatment of the AIS patient.

The addition of perfusion techniques to conventional CT or MR scanning achieves a better patient selection and the appropriate choice of therapy for the individual patient (no treatment versus rescue treatment or reperfusion).[27,28]

Evidence shows that identification of the tissue at risk for ischemia, known as penumbra, and its quantification make for a better choice of patients and appropriate therapy plan regarding each case.

Tissue at risk, also called penumbra area, is defined as a tissue area where perfusion is severely decreased; it can eventually become part of the core if reperfusion is absent.[29,30]

Several authors have pointed out the usefulness of perfusion (CTP or MRP, according to the technique) for the assessment of brain tissue, because perfusion can differentiate between ischemic infarcted tissue which is not salvageable and tissue impaired regarding circulation and function but still viable.

Some authors have proposed the use of perfusion CT images to define the margin of the infarct core, although no evidence supports the accuracy of that information.[23,29,31,32]

It is a fact that there are no significant differences between core size as assessed by perfusion CT and the one reached by the use of the ASPECTS score.[33]

Some years ago a concept came into use for the differentiation of those compromised areas after occlusion; it was the mismatch between non-contrast CT and MR perfusion mapping (DWI).

Two areas of affected tissue are then to be distinguished: the core, that is to say the center of the infarct where cytotoxic edema is to be found, and the hypoperfused periphery, known as penumbra zone.

Within the infarct core loss of blood flow is complete and lasting, and the breakdown of self-regulatory mechanisms is likewise permanent. Consequently, both CBF and CBV are decreased. (▶ Fig. 4.8)

On the other hand, only CBF is decreased in the penumbra zone because self-regulation keeps CBV within normal limits or even allows for its increase.

In both zones MTT is increased because contrast medium circulates with difficulty through the capillary bed of the compromised tissue. (▶ Fig. 4.9).

The best-known method is CTP, and also the one most frequently used. In spite of its being very much in use in several centers, it is not frequently included as a criterion for the choice of patients.

On the other hand, two big and well-known studies (DEFUSE and EPITHET) have evidenced the importance of detecting penumbra and using it as a parameter for the choice of patients.[34]

The combination of mismatch and early reperfusion after thrombolysis is associated to a better neurological outcome.[34]

There is some lack of agreement in scientific literature about the definition of mismatch between necrotic zone and hypoperfused zone. The difference between them is the crucial factor at the moment of making a decision.

In this respect, the reference value of CBF for the infarct core is under 40–50% of the values of the contralateral tissue, or if absolute values are taken, 2.0–2.2 ml/100 g.

For the penumbra at-risk tissue MTT is increased 145% over the reference value in the contralateral tissue, which serves to differentiate it from benign oligemia. The latter is defined as hypoperfused tissue that is not threatened by ischemia like the actual penumbra zone.

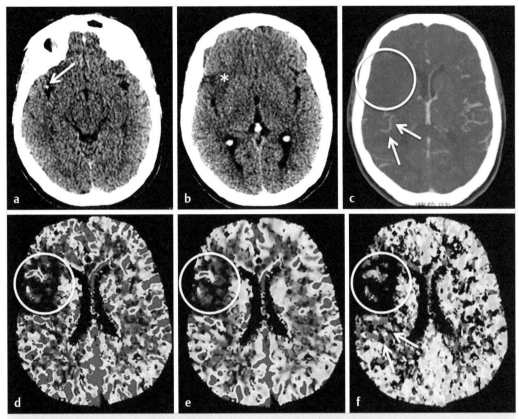

Fig. 4.8 Multimodal CT in hyperacute ischemic stroke (mismatch). Patient with focal neurological impairment beginning 70 minutes ago. **(a, b)** Non-contrast CT shows hyperdense middle cerebral artery sign (arrow) and hypodensity limited to the insula (*). **(c)** Angio-CT images evidence the area of impaired flow (inside the dotted line) and the presence of collaterals distal to it (arrow). **(d-f)** CT perfusion studies consist of the CBV map at **(d)**, the CBF map at **(e)** and the MTT map at **(f)**. The area mentioned above evidences decreased CBV and MTT, while in the zone distal to it CBV is preserved and MTT is increased (arrows). This latter area corresponds to the potentially salvageable tissue known as penumbra.

The significance of ischemic tissue quantification has been confirmed. Not so the importance of ischemic tissue volume, a factor whose incidence on prognosis is still under discussion. Even if revascularization is adequate, recovery of capillary circulation may not modify perfusion parameters significantly.

That is why the impact of quantification on the prognosis of penumbra is debatable, and the usefulness of these techniques for patient selection is also questionable.

In AIS patients, the clinical impact of perfusion techniques on the progress of the disease and above all, its importance for decision making, has not been demonstrated at acceptable levels of evidence. Several studies (DEFUSE, DEFUSE-2, EPI-THET) have shown that these techniques hold promise to identify candidates for late revascularization therapy. Meanwhile other studies like MR-RESCUE, for example, have shown no benefit at all.

Another interesting point is the correlation between DWI/ADC findings and NIHSS score for the clinical estimation of penumbra. Regarding this question, several authors do not use perfusion techniques for the quantification of at-risk tissue.[1,35]

A recent meta-analysis suggests that perfusion techniques may be considered a complementary tool for the selection of patients for reperfusion therapy, in spite of their limitations.[30]

According to present evidence, it is not appropriate to exclude patients from recanalization treatments, using cerebral perfusion as the main parameter. But in particular situations like a stroke

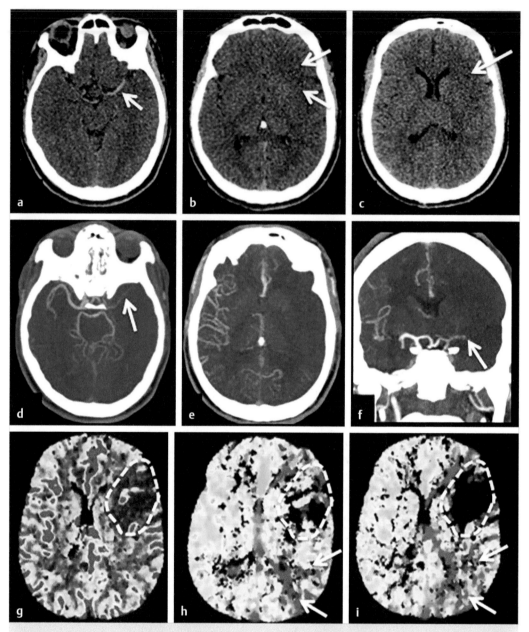

Fig. 4.9 Multimodal CT in hyperacute stroke (mismatch). (a-c) Non-contrast CT scans of a patient who presented with right hemiplegia dating from 3 hours ago. Hyperdense middle cerebral artery sign **(a)**, effacement of anterior sector of insula **(b)** and effacement of anterior frontal lobe **(c)**. **(d-f)** Angio-CT scans show proximal occlusion of left MCA (arrow) and the absence of collaterals distal to it. **(g-i)** Perfusion studies show an area of decreased CBV at **(g)** and an extensive penumbra zone, evidenced by increased MTT, at the territory distal to the MCA **(h, i)**

of uncertain onset or a patient outside the therapeutic window, cerebral perfusion may be taken into consideration.

4.6 AIS of Uncertain Onset

As was previously mentioned, one of the most important parameters in the strategy of decision-making is the time from onset. At the hyperacute stage (up to 4.5 hours from clinical onset) both the contribution of imaging methods and their impact on the choice of treatment have been clearly established.

In a not inconsiderable percentage of cases the time of onset is not clear. For example, AIS on awakening (which accounts for up to 25% of cases according to some series) presents in this way.

A few years ago this uncertainty excluded the patient from all possible reperfusion therapies, no matter the method.

Taking into account an improved understanding of physiology and its alterations during cerebral ischemia and also the information provided by different methods, it is now possible to better select these patients and assign them to the most adequate protocol.

Using unrestricted protocols, above all MR protocols, it is possible to estimate the volume of tissue at risk for ischemia if adequate reperfusion is not attained.[36]

Several authors have reported that these patients may be included in the therapeutic algorithm if no evidence of ischemia appears in the FLAIR sequence on the MR scans.[37]

The concept of mismatch arises in this context, but in this case as the difference between zones of ischemia and zones of penumbra in the DWI/ADC and FLAIR sequences.[20] (▶ Fig. 4.10, ▶ Fig. 4.11)

As previously mentioned the DWI/ADC sequence is the most sensitive for early ischemic changes while the FLAIR changes set in later.[38] Therefore, the difference in compromised tissue between the two sequences represents the area with very early ischemia. This concept, which is quite specific for cases dating where clinical impairment began 3 to 4,5 hours before, permits recruiting those patients in the protocol most suitable for their needs.

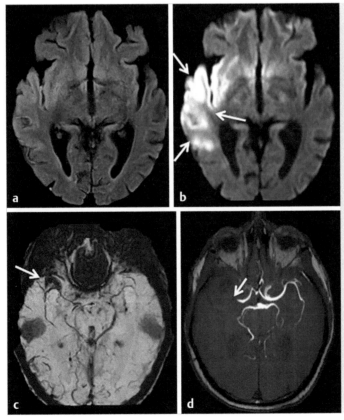

Fig. 4.10 Stroke of uncertain onset, DWI/FLAIR mismatch. (a) Normal FLAIR sequence in a patient who awoke hemiparetic on his left side. **(b)** DWI scans of the same patient, showing cytotoxic edema in the right MCA territory (arrows). **(c, d)** SWI scan in **(c)**, with evidence of a proximal thrombus at the homolateral MCA (arrow), and an equivalent zone in the axial plane of the TOF sequence of the angio-MR in **(d)** (arrow).

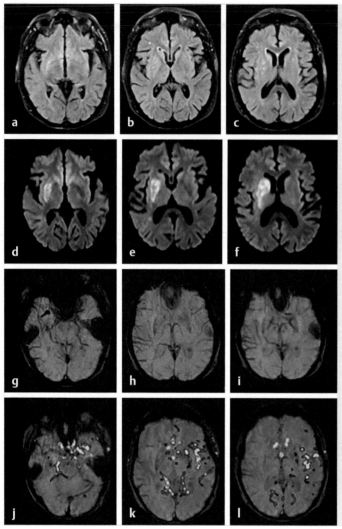

Fig. 4.11 Stroke of uncertain onset, Multimodal MR. Multimodal MR study of patient found lying on the floor, evidencing left hemiplegia. **(a-c)** No significant alterations in the FLAIR sequence. **(d-f)** DWI sequence shows cytotoxic edema in the deep territory of the right MCA. **(g-i)** SWI scans evidencing proximal thrombus at **(g)**, slowing of distal flow at **(h, i)**, indicating perfusion impairment and determining the penumbra area (DWI/FLAIR mismatch).**(j-l)** Perfusion scan with ASL technique shows impaired cerebral blood flow in the territory of the right MCA.

4.7 Finals Concepts

The considerable change in the therapeutic approach to AIS patients in the last few years is fundamentally due not only to advances in endovascular treatment but also to a better understanding of the alterations occurring in brain parenchyma.

This is where advanced imaging methods have contributed basic information that permitted the development of different strategic approaches to the AIS patient at the hyperacute stage.

These methods show high sensitivity and specificity for the exclusion of hemorrhage; are able to identify and quantify the infarct core; are capable of analyzing potentially at-risk tissue (penumbra zone), and can locate vascular occlusion very precisely. All these factors have had significant impact in the choice of the best therapeutic approach for the individual patient.

Both multimodal CT and advanced MR provide sufficient information for an adequate therapeutic approach.[39] The method must be chosen taking into account local factors, which includes not only available equipment but training and experience of the techniques en each center. Above all, the chosen method must include the highest number of patients within the therapeutic window.[40]

We think that MR, in spite of its logistic limitations, is the method that selects a bigger group of suitable patients and therefore has a more significant impact on survival and functional prognosis.

References

[1] González RG, Copen WA, Schaefer PW, et al. The Massachusetts General Hospital acute stroke imaging algorithm: an experience and evidence based approach. J Neurointerv Surg. 2013; 5 Suppl 1:i7–i12

[2] Latchaw RE, Alberts MJ, Lev MH, et al. American Heart Association Council on Cardiovascular Radiology and Intervention, Stroke Council, and the Interdisciplinary Council on Peripheral Vascular Disease. Recommendations for imaging of acute ischemic stroke: a scientific statement from the American Heart Association. Stroke. 2009; 40(11):3646–3678

[3] Demchuk AM, Hill MD, Barber PA, Silver B, Patel SC, Levine SR, NINDS rtPA Stroke Study Group, NIH. Importance of early ischemic computed tomography changes using ASPECTS in NINDS rtPA Stroke Study. Stroke. 2005; 36(10):2110–2115

[4] Bouchez L, Sztajzel R, Vargas MI, et al. CT imaging selection in acute stroke. Eur J Radiol. 2016

[5] Berkhemer OA, Fransen PS, Beumer D, et al. MR CLEAN Investigators. A randomized trial of intraarterial treatment for acute ischemic stroke. N Engl J Med. 2015; 372(1):11–20

[6] Menon BK, Goyal M. Imaging Paradigms in Acute Ischemic Stroke: A Pragmatic Evidence-based Approach. Radiology. 2015; 277(1):7–12

[7] Nael K, Kubal W. Magnetic Resonance Imaging of Acute Stroke. Magn Reson Imaging Clin N Am. 2016; 24(2):293–304

[8] González RG, Schaefer PW, Buonanno FS, et al. Diffusion-weighted MR imaging: diagnostic accuracy in patients imaged within 6 hours of stroke symptom onset. Radiology. 1999; 210(1):155–162

[9] Grigoryan M, Tung CE, Albers GW. Role of diffusion and perfusion MRI in selecting patients for reperfusion therapies. Neuroimaging Clin N Am. 2011; 21(2):247–257, ix–x

[10] Lövblad KO, Altrichter S, Mendes Pereira V, et al. Imaging of acute stroke: CT and/or MRI. J Neuroradiol. 2015; 42(1):55–64

[11] Hill MD, Demchuk AM, Tomsick TA, Palesch YY, Broderick JP. Using the baseline CT scan to select acute stroke patients for IV-IA therapy. AJNR Am J Neuroradiol. 2006; 27(8):1612–1616

[12] Jauch EC, Saver JL, Adams HP, Jr, et al. American Heart Association Stroke Council, Council on Cardiovascular Nursing, Council on Peripheral Vascular Disease, Council on Clinical Cardiology. Guidelines for the early management of patients with acute ischemic stroke: a guideline for healthcare professionals from the American Heart Association/American Stroke Association. Stroke. 2013; 44(3):870–947

[13] von Kummer R, Early CT. Early CT Score to establish stroke treatment. Lancet Neurol. 2016; 15(7):651–653

[14] von Kummer R, Dzialowski I, Gerber J. Therapeutic efficacy of brain imaging in acute ischemic stroke patients. J Neuroradiol. 2015; 42(1):47–54

[15] Schellinger PD, Bryan RN, Caplan LR, et al. Therapeutics and Technology Assessment Subcommittee of the American Academy of Neurology. Evidence-based guideline: The role of diffusion and perfusion MRI for the diagnosis of acute ischemic stroke: report of the Therapeutics and Technology Assessment Subcommittee of the American Academy of Neurology. Neurology. 2010; 75(2):177–185

[16] Yaghi S, Bianchi N, Amole A, Hinduja A. ASPECTS is a predictor of favorable CT perfusion in acute ischemic stroke. J Neuroradiol. 2014; 41(3):184–187

[17] González RG. Current state of acute stroke imaging. Stroke. 2013; 44(11):3260–3264

[18] Wolf RL, Alsop DC, McGarvey ML, Maldjian JA, Wang J, Detre JA. Susceptibility contrast and arterial spin labeled perfusion MRI in cerebrovascular disease. J Neuroimaging. 2003; 13(1):17–27

[19] Yoo AJ, Verduzco LA, Schaefer PW, Hirsch JA, Rabinov JD, González RG. MRI-based selection for intra-arterial stroke therapy: value of pretreatment diffusion-weighted imaging lesion volume in selecting patients with acute stroke who will benefit from early recanalization. Stroke. 2009; 40(6):2046–2054

[20] Lansberg MG, Straka M, Kemp S, et al. DEFUSE 2 study investigators. MRI profile and response to endovascular reperfusion after stroke (DEFUSE 2): a prospective cohort study. Lancet Neurol. 2012; 11(10):860–867

[21] Tomanek AI, Coutts SB, Demchuk AM, et al. MR angiography compared to conventional selective angiography in acute stroke. Can J Neurol Sci. 2006; 33(1):58–62

[22] Yoo AJ, Barak ER, Copen WA, et al. Combining acute diffusion-weighted imaging and mean transmit time lesion volumes with National Institutes of Health Stroke Scale Score improves the prediction of acute stroke outcome. Stroke. 2010; 41(8):1728–1735

[23] González RG, Lev MH, Goldmacher GV, et al. Improved outcome prediction using CT angiography in addition to standard ischemic stroke assessment: results from the STOPStroke study. PLoS One. 2012; 7(1):e30352

[24] Varadharajan S, Saini J, Acharya UV, Gupta AK. Computed tomography angiography in acute stroke (revisiting the 4Ps of imaging). Am J Emerg Med. 2016; 34(2):282–287

[25] Lev MH, Farkas J, Rodríguez VR, et al. CT angiography in the rapid triage of patients with hyperacute stroke to intraarterial thrombolysis: accuracy in the detection of large vessel thrombus. J Comput Assist Tomogr. 2001; 25(4):520–528

[26] Bash S, Villablanca JP, Jahan R, et al. Intracranial vascular stenosis and occlusive disease: evaluation with CT angiography, MR angiography, and digital subtraction angiography. AJNR Am J Neuroradiol. 2005; 26(5):1012–1021

[27] Kawano H, Bivard A, Lin L, et al. Perfusion computed tomography in patients with stroke thrombolysis. Brain. 2017; 140(3):684–691

[28] Campbell BC, Mitchell PJ, Kleinig TJ, et al. EXTEND-IA Investigators. Endovascular therapy for ischemic stroke with perfusion-imaging selection. N Engl J Med. 2015; 372(11):1009–1018

[29] Bivard A, Levi C, Krishnamurthy V, et al. Defining acute ischemic stroke tissue pathophysiology with whole brain CT perfusion. J Neuroradiol. 2014; 41(5):307–315

[30] Ryu WHA, Avery MB, Dharampal N, Allen IE, Hetts SW. Utility of perfusion imaging in acute stroke treatment: a systematic review and meta-analysis. J Neurointerv Surg. 2017; 9(10):1012–1016

[31] Aviv RI, Mandelcorn J, Chakraborty S, et al. Alberta Stroke Program Early CT Scoring of CT perfusion in early stroke visualization and assessment. AJNR Am J Neuroradiol. 2007; 28(10):1975–1980

[32] Baron JC. Mapping the ischaemic penumbra with PET: implications for acute stroke treatment. Cerebrovasc Dis. 1999; 9(4):193–201

[33] Fung SH, Roccatagliata L, Gonzalez RG, Schaefer PW. MR diffusion imaging in ischemic stroke. Neuroimaging Clin N Am. 2011; 21(2):345–377, xi

[34] Albers GW, Thijs VN, Wechsler L, et al. DEFUSE Investigators. Magnetic resonance imaging profiles predict clinical response to early reperfusion: the diffusion and perfusion imaging evaluation for understanding stroke evolution (DEFUSE) study. Ann Neurol. 2006; 60(5):508–517

[35] Deb P, Sharma S, Hassan KM. Pathophysiologic mechanisms of acute ischemic stroke: An overview with emphasis on therapeutic significance beyond thrombolysis. Pathophysiology. 2010; 17(3):197–218

[36] Petkova M, Rodrigo S, Lamy C, et al. MR imaging helps predict time from symptom onset in patients with acute stroke: implications for patients with unknown onset time. Radiology. 2010; 257(3):782–792

[37] Nagai K, Aoki J, Sakamoto Y, Kimura K. About 30% of wake-up stroke patients may be candidate for the tPA therapy using Negative-FLAIR as a "tissue clock". J Neurol Sci. 2017; 382:101–104

[38] Aoki J, Kimura K, Iguchi Y, Shibazaki K, Sakai K, Iwanaga T. FLAIR can estimate the onset time in acute ischemic stroke patients. J Neurol Sci. 2010; 293(1–2):39–44

[39] Vo KD, Yoo AJ, Gupta A, et al. Multimodal Diagnostic Imaging for Hyperacute Stroke. AJNR Am J Neuroradiol. 2015; 36(12): 2206–2213

[40] Vymazal J, Rulseh AM, Keller J, Janouskova L. Comparison of CT and MR imaging in ischemic stroke. Insights Imaging. 2012; 3(6):619–627

5 Neurosurgical Treatment for Hemorrhagic and Ischemic Stroke

Behnam Rezai Jahromi, Akitsugu Kawashima, Joham Choque-Velasquez, Christopher Ludtka Beng, Danil A. Kozyrev, Felix Göhre, and Juha Hernesniemi

Abstract

Hemorrhagic and ischemic strokes have significant global burden and correct diagnosis and treatment requires co-operation of units of society at large as time window for treating these lesion is narrow. Neurosurgeons' role varies by country and department when it is about ischemic stroke but is fairly dominant in hemorrhagic strokes. Treatment of vascular anomalies such as aneurysms, arteriovenous malformations, and moyamoya disease are described in this chapter. Also intracerebral hematomas which some times requires surgical intervention.

Keywords: aneurysm, arteriovenous malformation, bypass surgery, intracerebral hematomas, revascularization, moyamoya

5.1 Historical Role of Neurosurgery for Stroke

A stroke is a sudden critical function failure of the brain, which can result from ischemic causes or intracranial bleeding. The clinical implications regarding diagnosis and treatment are common to both types of stroke, ischemic and hemorrhagic. The aim of any treatment is the prevention of secondary brain damage. However, ischemic stroke is one of the most common causes of death worldwide and one of the main sources of disability. Stroke prevention and modern stroke treatment have decreased incidence and mortality in western countries during the last few decades. In spite of this progress, the expected demographic shift due to an aging population will only heighten the importance of ischemic stroke management in coming years. Neurosurgical treatment options are required in all stroke units. Particularly so since the cause of stroke is initially unknown and the occurrence of secondary bleeding complications is always possible. Aneurysms, AVMs, hematoma evacuation, and cerebral revascularization, including moyamoya, are summarized below. Many important stroke-related neurosurgical procedures are the subject of other chapters (e.g. decompressive craniectomy).

5.2 Surgery for Acute Hemorrhagic Stroke or Intracerebral Hematomas

Primary intracerebral hemorrhages occur in approximately 10% of strokes. The most common causes of hemorrhagic strokes are: hypertension (30–60%), cerebral amyloid angiopathy (10–30%), anticoagulation (1–20%), and vascular structural lesions (3–8%); idiopathic stroke comprises 5–20% of cases. Supratentorial intracerebral hemorrhages account for 85–95% of cases. Within this group, lobar hemorrhages represent 25–40% of cases, and deep brain structure hemorrhages 50–75%. The 30-day mortality is higher for deep hemorrhages than for lobar ones, and mortality rises with hemorrhage volume. Intracerebral hemorrhages may be associated with various complications such as rebleeding with expansion of the hematoma, hydrocephalus, intraventricular hemorrhage, and edema. Patients with a cerebellar hematoma are at particular risk of deterioration, specifically due to direct compression of the brainstem and cerebellum. The risk of hematoma expansion and hydrocephalus underlines the importance of careful neurological monitoring and 24-hour access to computed tomography scanning in cases of deterioration. Early surgical evacuation of supratentorial hematomas might be beneficial for patients with a Glasgow Coma Scale score of 9–12 who are treated within 8 hours after symptom onset. A minimally invasive drainage via catheter may represent a promising treatment option for deep hematomas. An external ventricular drain combined with topical fibrinolysis may reduce mortality, though it does not seem to be related to better functional outcomes in patients with intraventricular hemorrhage and hydrocephalus. Surgical evacuation of infratentorial intracerebral hemorrhages is typically indicated if the Glasgow Coma Scale score is lower than 14, the hematoma diameter greater than 30–40 mm, the hematoma volume greater than 7 cm^3, or if there is an obliteration of the fourth ventricle. An external ventricular drain is usually inserted if there is an associated hydrocephalus.

General recommendations to manage hemorrhagic stroke include: (7)

- Stroke services should agree upon and share protocols for the monitoring, referral, and transfer of patients to regional neurosurgical centers for the management of symptomatic hydrocephalus.
- Patients with intracranial hemorrhages should be monitored in neurosurgical or stroke care for deterioration in function, and referred immediately for brain imaging when necessary.
- Previously healthy patients should be considered for surgical intervention if the intracranial hemorrhage causes hydrocephalus.
- Patients with any of the following conditions rarely require surgical intervention and should receive medical treatment initially: small deep hemorrhages; lobar hemorrhages with neither hydrocephalus nor rapid neurological deterioration; a large intracerebral hemorrhage and concurrent with significant prior co-morbidities; a Glasgow Coma Scale (GCS) score below 8, unless due to hydrocephalus.

5.3 Aneurysm and Stroke

Unruptured intracranial aneurysms (UIA) presenting with ischemic events such as transient ischemic attacks (TIAs) or ischemic stroke are relatively rare. The number of patients with cerebral aneurysms who presented with TIAs and/or stroke amounts to 0.5–6.6%. Ischemic episodes in patients with intracranial aneurysms are caused by thrombosed aneurysms or occlusion of the parent vessel. Several reports have shown that no matter how small the aneurysm, a thrombotic mass can migrate from its dome to the distal region of symptomatic cerebral arteries or spread to the parent artery.

5.3.1 Pathophysiology

There are mainly two reasons for intra-aneurysmal thrombus formation. First, the flow pattern inside of the aneurysm can stimulate thrombus formation. Second, the aneurysmal lumen can stimulate thrombosis. Both of these causes of thrombus formation also play a role in aneurysmal wall pathophysiology. Additionally, there is the possibility for thrombosis to increase via neovascularization or growth of the aneurysm. Likewise, in large and giant aneurysms (▶ Fig. 5.1), intramural hemorrhages due to rupture of fragile vasa vasorum stimulate thrombus formation. The dynamics of thrombus formation and lysis result in the appearance of emboli, which subsequently makes stroke inevitable. Unfortunately the thrombus inside the aneurysm does not protect the patient from aneurysm rupture, but can actually advance it. It is complete obliteration of an aneurysm and thrombotic

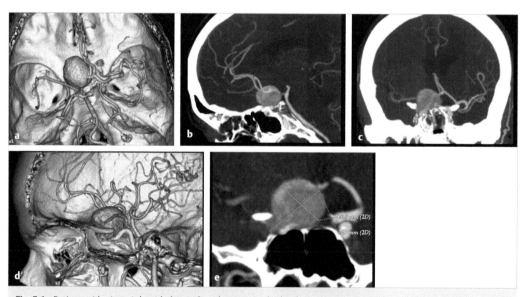

Fig. 5.1 Patient with giant right-sided paraclinoid aneurysm had ischemic symptoms. Diagnosis was made after TIA via MRI imaging. Aneurysm was treated by clip ligation.

mass removal that protect the patient from stroke. This is why open microneurosurgery is preferred. In many cases revascularization is necessary for such large and giant aneurysms. This should be done in medical centers dedicated to neurovascular treatment.

5.3.2 Treatment

Conservative Treatment

The management of unruptured aneurysms presenting with ischemic events does not have any consensus yet. However, signs of stroke and ischemia with unruptured aneurysms have been seen as indicatorions for treating these aneurysms. Since pathophysiology of aneurysms is largely dependent on thrombus formation. Rupture of aneurysm is stimulated by biological activity of thrombus.

Surgical and Endovascular Treatment

UIAs presenting with ischemic events are best treated by means of a microneurosurgical operation, a revascularization procedure consisting of the removal of potentially thrombotic and/or diseased segments of the arterial system. When comparing microneurosurgery to endovascular treatment, it is important to note that in many cases endovascular treatment is difficult due to thrombotic activity of endovascular devices and recanalization of the aneurysms. Surgical clipping brings healthy parts of the artery together and makes possible to endothelial section to heal. The mass effect of large and giant aneurysms is another contributing factor in the development of stroke. A stroke occurs through the mechanisms of perforating vessels occlusion and/or distal embolic events from thrombosed or partially-thrombosed aneurysm. Endovascular treatment may reduce the mass effect, as aneurysms usually decrease in size, but only surgical intervention can totally eliminate it. When anatomy allows, an aneurysm may be removed with or without preservation of blood flow in the involved vessel. This completely eradicates mass effect caused by an aneurysm and releases the surrounding structure from compression. Nevertheless, the surgical treatment of large and giant aneurysms remains one of the most challenging areas in vascular neurosurgery. These pathologies necessitate extensive experience in dealing with intracranial aneurysms. At the same time, endovascular treatment has reached meaningful success but still cannot totally replace open surgical intervention.

5.3.3 Conclusion

The outcome of patients harboring unruptured intracranial aneurysms and presenting with TIAs and ischemic stroke has improved during the last few decades. Only complete exclusion of an aneurysm can guarantee prevention of recurrent TIAs and stroke caused by the aneurysm. However, treatment of complex aneurysms should be done in high-volume centers specifically dedicated to these difficult lesions. In many cases, the same patients suffer from co-morbidities (e.g. diabetes, atherosclerosis, cardiac diseases) and therefore require further medical treatment to prevent excess mortality.

5.4 Arteriovenous Malformation and Stroke

Most patients with cerebral arteriovenous malformation (AVM) are diagnosed during middle-age, meaning that they have potentially decades of life ahead. Helsinki study of the natural history of AVMs is in line with the ARUBA study (A Randomized trial of Unruptured Brain AVMs): there exists an approximately 2–3% annual risk of hemorrhage. The indications for treating these lesions are easy to understand and readily justified. The collective risk of rupture of AVMs will grow significantly over the span of a patient's life and the only way to avoid such a hemorrhage is to remove the AVM. Originally, ARUBA investigators came to conclude that conservative treatment is superior to intervention at 33 months follow-up. Regrettably, the same investigators later extrapolated that the results of ARUBA were valid as follow-up data decades later. Fortunately for patients, the neurovascular community has woken up from this disastrous way of thinking and there are now many other studies which report more rational conclusions for patient care. No one can know the obliteration rate of AVMs in the ARUBA study, as it has not been reported. More than half of the intervention group either had on-going treatment or had not started treatment (53 and 20 patients, respectively) during the report of ARUBA. Meta-analysis by Liu X showed that 96% of AVMs are removable by microneurosurgery, 38% by radiation, and 13% by embolization. Despite this knowledge, only 17 patients out of 114 in the ARUBA intervention group were treated by micro-neurosurgery, even though 76 patients in the intervention group had Spetzler-Martin (SM) Grade I-II. Additionally, approximately one-third of patients in the ARUBA study were SM grade III-IV; as such this subgroup is overrepresented in the patient cohort. Obviously intervention in such cases is riskier than for lower grade AVMs. All this shows that complex diseases such as AVMs should be treated in medical centers dedicated to them by professionals who treat these lesions daily.

5.5 Cerebral Revascularization

5.5.1 Microsurgical Embolectomy

Embolic occlusion of a major intracranial vessel is a life-threatening event. Therefore, active treatment within a narrowed time window is necessary for a favorable outcome. Intra-venous or intra-arterial thrombolysis and endovascular mechanical embolectomy have been considered the best options to date. However microsurgical embolectomies represent a safe treatment method with

high revascularization rates in very experienced hands. Since Welch reported the first surgical embolectomy of an intracranial vessel in 1956 several promising reports of successful microsurgical embolectomies with high recanalization rates have been published. The focused opening and microsurgical dissection of the Sylvian fissure is now a standard neurosurgical procedure. Exposure of the whole affected segment is required to obtain complete vessel control. Temporary occlusion of all side branches avoids further embolism into these branches. A transverse arteriotomy allows for the evacuation of the embolus and can subsequently be sutured (▶ Fig. 5.2) The described technique can be applied to other intracranial bifurcations (ICAbif and MCAbif) as typical predilection sides for embolic occlusions. However, the indication is based on an individual treatment approach under consideration of the general stroke guidelines.

5.5.2 Cerebral Bypass Surgeries

Several kinds of pathologies of the brain can be managed by revascularization of the arterial system. Mainly these lesions are aneurysms (large,

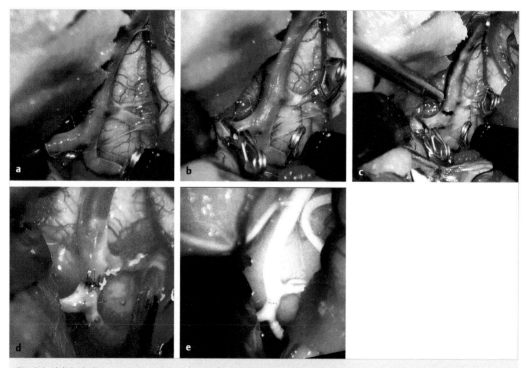

Fig. 5.2 (a) Embolus seen in artery (media cerebral artery, M2 section) as blue colored mass intraluminally. (b) Temporal clips are used distal of the thrombus. (c) Small incision is made in the artery. (d) Thrombus is removed. (e) ICG shows recanalization of the artery.

dolichoectatic, or fusiform), abnormal network in moya moya disease, and certain tumors.

In this part of the chapter we concentrate on vascular lesions, which can induce stroke or have already shown signs of stroke and are in need of revascularization. Generally revascularization can be divided to two categories; extracranial-to-intracranial (EC-IC) and intracranial-to-intracranial (IC-IC) bypasses.

Anatomical possibilities of some of the most common revascularization procedures are:
- EC-IC
  - Superior temporal artery (STA) to middle cerebral artery
  - STA to posterior cerebral artery
  - STA to superior cerebral artery
- IC-IC
  - Occipital artery (OA) to anterior inferior cerebellar artery
  - OA to posterior inferior cerebellar artery
  - PICA to PICA
- Graft to EC or/and IC
  - Individualized treatment for complex aneurysms
  - Graft can be radial artery or saphenous vein

The aim of this section is to encourage readers to accumulate more information and technical aspects on complex aneurysms. Many aneurysms are treatable in experienced units whom have concentrated on complex neurovascular procedures.

Bypass Surgeries Applied to the Anterior Cerebral Circulation

The main idea of anterior circulation revascularization is showed in moyamoya section of the chapter.

Bypass Surgeries Applied to the Posterior Cerebral Circulation

Atherosclerotic occlusive disease is the major reason for hemodynamic impairment of the posterior circulation. Posterior circulation stroke can present various symptoms such as: dizziness, nausea, cranial nerve palsy, swallowing difficulties, eye movement disturbance, isolated homonymous hemianopia, motor and sensory deficits, and loss of consciousness. Direct surgical revascularization is technically demanding and is reserved for selected cases based on individualized indications. However, bypass bridging techniques are well-documented and effective for the treatment of hemodynamic insufficiency affecting the posterior

circulation. The upper posterior circulation can by revascularized by using the superficial temporal artery as a donor vessel and the superior cerebellar artery or posterior cerebral artery as recipient. The lower posterior circulation can be revascularized using an occipital artery to posterior inferior cerebellar artery bypass. An uncommon cause of posterior circulation stroke is rotational vertebral artery compression syndrome. The disease is usually aggravated by its dynamic component. The dynamic conventional angiography is the gold standard of imaging. However, the treatment of patients with rotational vertebral artery compression syndrome requires an individual approach. Conservative treatment includes neck immobilization and anticoagulant therapy. Surgical treatment requires operative decompression in cases of external stenosis by osteophytes and fixation by segmental fusion in cases of instability.

5.5.3 Moyamoya Disease

Definition of MMD

Moyamoya disease (MMD) is characterized by progressive occlusion at bilateral internal carotid artery (ICA) terminals, resulting in poor vascularity with the development of an abnormal vascular network. Histopathological features of MMD are fibrocellular thickening of the intima, waving of the internal elastic lamina, and attenuation of the media in the carotid terminations, all of which make itis different from intracranial atherosclerotic disease (ICAD). According to the guideline for diagnosis and treatment of moyamoya disease, cases with unilateral lesion are categorized as unilateral MMD. MMD with conditions such as autoimmune disease, meningitis, von Recklinghausen's disease, brain tumor, Down's syndrome, hyperthyroidism, sickle cell disease, etc. are categorized as quasi-MMD. Arteriosclerotic disease and patients with a history of radiation therapy are defined as non-MMD.

5.5.4 Surgical Management

1. Revascularization for ischemic MMD: indication, timing, surgical procedures, and perioperative management

The most important indication for MMD revascularization is previous cerebral ischemia, as this will improve with a new hemodynamic pattern. Revascularization is done for patients with ischemic symptoms and ischemic evidence by SPECT/Xe CT/

PET imaging. For pediatric patients however, cerebral revascularization is occasionally considered even without typical ischemic symptoms. Cerebral ischemia can be progressive in some MMD patients. Ischemic symptoms, which are sometimes unclear, include: headache, involuntary movements, syncope, numbness, dizziness, etc. Surgical procedures are divided into direct and indirect revascularization. Superficial temporal artery (STA) to middle cerebral artery (MCA) bypass has been established as the direct bypass procedure for MMD. Direct bypass can lead to immediate improvement of symptoms, however it is also technically demanding. Meta-analysis shows that direct bypass, including the combined approach, is superior to indirect revascularization for future stroke prevention and angiographic outcome. Regarding perioperative complications, there are no differences between direct bypass and indirect revascularization. Furthermore, direct bypass using the STA graft is applicable for revascularization not only in the MCA territory but also in the anterior cerebral artery territory. Anti-platelet therapy is generally considered for patients with an acute ischemic state. A latency period of 2–3 weeks after the last ischemic attack is required before revascularization. However, timing of revascularization surgery for patients who suffer from progressive stroke is controversial.

- Direct bypass is sometimes considered in the subacute stage for progressive stroke patients;
- Oral administration of 100 mg acetylsalicylic acid (ASA) is recommended for treatment of acute phase of ischemic stroke;
- and support of revascularization for in patients of in the chronic ischemic phase.

ASA treatment is started 7 days prior to operation, and it is continued for several months postoperatively

- except for a pause of 3 days after the operation. Systolic blood pressure should stay strictly under control, going no further than 100 mmHg to 140 mmHg after operation to prevent ischemic stroke and hyperperfusion syndrome. Arterial carbon dioxide (paCO2) should be remain around 40 mmHg during and after operation.

Revascularization for Hemorrhagic MMD

Half of adult MMD patients present with intracranial hemorrhage, which dramatically worsens the prognosis and causes a high rebleeding rate. Hemorrhage is usually caused by tiny, fragile collateral vessels: so-called moyamoya vessels. Direct bypass is considered supposed to decrease the hemodynamic stress on moyamoya vessels. According to the Japan Adult Moyamoya (JAM) trial, direct bypass for adult MMD patients is proven to reduce rebleeding rate and improve the patient's prognosis. Subgroup analysis of JAM trial reveals that patients with posterior site hemorrhage are at higher risk of rebleeding and direct bypass provides greater benefits compared to those attained in patients with anterior site hemorrhage.

Case Presentation

A 37-year-old woman presented with a small, right thalamic hemorrhage 4 years ago. She had also suffered from repeated transient symptoms of bilateral numbness and slight motor weakness for several years. MRI demonstrated a hemorrhage scar in the right thalamus and an old infarction in the right water shed area. MRA showed occlusion/severe stenosis in the bilateral ICA terminal and the right P1 with moyamoya vessels. (▶ Fig. 5.3 **a**) SPECT showed a severe decrease in cerebral blood flow (CBF) with cerebrovascular reactivity (CVR) in the right whole territory and the left MCA territory. (▶ Fig. 5.3 **b**) The patient underwent right STA-MCA double bypass. (▶ Fig. 5.4 **a, b**) Postoperative SPECT showed severe hyperperfusion in the subcortical frontal region just around the anastomosis. (▶ Fig. 5.4 **c**) Patient was kept under sedation until the next morning, her systolic blood pressure kept strictly under control, going no further than 100–120 mmHg. Her postoperative condition was good except for transient dysarthria on day 6, post-op. One year after the first operation, left STA-MCA double bypass was performed. MRA 6 months after the second operation demonstrated decreasing of moyamoya vessels bilaterally and good blood supply from both grafts. (▶ Fig. 5.5 **a**) Post-operative SPECT revealed hyperperfusion, but this occurrence did not affect the patient's postoperative condition. CBF and CVR in both hemispheres were significantly improved in SPECT 6 months after second operation. (▶ Fig. 5.5 **b**) Angiography before (▶ Fig. 5.6 **a**) and 6 months after second operation (▶ Fig. 5.6 **b,c**) shows the source of blood supply to the cortical arteries shifting from the ICAs to the grafts with diminished moyamoya vessels.

Distinction Between MMD and ICAD

MMD is diagnosed based on radiological findings; this morphologic diagnosis, however, confuses the

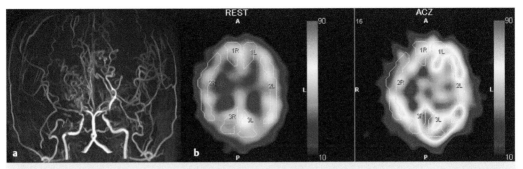

Fig. 5.3 **(a, b)** Intraoperative photos and **(c)**postoperative image. **(a)** The superficial temporal artery (STA) graft anastomosing to the M4 intermittently with 10–0 mono filament. Blue colored silicon stent inserting in the lumen of the M4 to prevent suturing the contralateral vessel wall. **(b)** Right STA-middle temporal cerebral artery double bypasses being made.

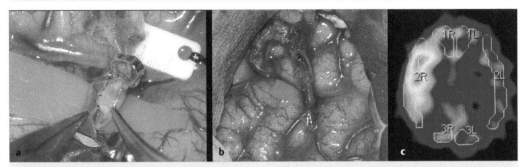

Fig. 5.4 Postoperative images 6 months after second operation. **(a)** MRA demonstrating decrease of moyamoya vessels bilaterally and extreme blood supply from both grafts. **(b)** SPECT showing marked improvement of cerebral blood flow and cerebrovascular reactivity in both hemispheres.

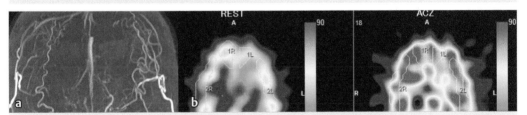

Fig. 5.5 **(a)** Preoperative, and **(b, c)** postoperative angiography. **(a)** Left internal carotid angiography before operation. Left internal carotid angiography **(b)** and left external angiography **(c)** 6 months after operation. Angiography showing source of blood supply to the cortical arteries appearing to shift from the internal carotid artery to the grafts with diminished moyamoya vessels.

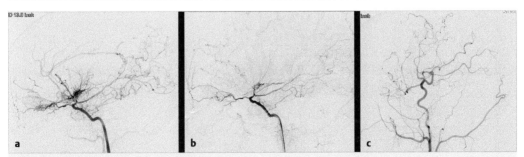

Fig. 5.6 **(a)** Embolus seen in artery (media cerebral artery, M2 section) as blue colored mass intraluminally. **(b)** Temporal clips are used distal of the thrombus. **(c)** Small incision is made in the artery. **(d)** Thrombus is removed. **(e)** ICG shows recanalization of the artery.

distinction between MMD and ICAD. Many times it is hard to distinguish MMD from ICAD. Recently, Kuroda et. al. provided a novel diagnosis method to distinguish MMD from ICAD. They analyzed the outer diameter of the stenotic vessels on three-dimensional constructive interference in steady state (3D-CISS) images according to the histopathological features of MMD. The outer diameter of the stenotic vessels around the ICA terminal in MMD patients was significantly smaller than the controls and in ICAD patients.

Postoperative Hyperperfusion

There are some specific postoperative complications of direct bypass for patients with MMD. One of the most severe postoperative complications is subcortical hemorrhage as a result of hyperperfusion. The mechanism of the postoperative hyperperfusion in patients with MMD is considered to be related to the vulnerability of the blood-brain barrier and is attributed to expanding capillary vessels, and increasing fragility of vessel walls over a long period of chronic ischemia. Transient focal neurological deficits present according to the specific lesion of the hyperperfusion, typically appearing 1–7 days after surgery. Subcortical hemorrhage or subarachnoid hemorrhage just around anastomosis could occur the day after operation, or occasionally several days after operation. The management of hyperperfusion is as important as brain ischemia. Intensive blood pressure control, prevention of convulsion, and sometimes deep sedation are recommended for patients with hyperperfusion. From personal experience (A. K.), the more developed the surgeon's skill regarding direct bypass, the greater the blood flow to be achieved in the graft and the less frequent the occurrence of hyperperfusion.

Cognitive Dysfunction

The progression of cognitive dysfunction in the natural course for MMD patients is unclear. Moreover, no adequate evidence has yet been provided to suggest the effectiveness of surgical revascularization in preventing and/or improving cognitive dysfunction. However, some studies have claimed that chronic hemodynamic disturbances are associated with cognitive dysfunction in patients with MMD, and that surgical revascularization has the potential to reverse cognitive dysfunction caused by hemodynamic impairment. It is essential to establish evaluation criteria for patients with cognitive dysfunction to determine which patients would benefit from surgical revascularization. It is expected that surgical revascularization can be proven to prevent and/or improve cognitive dysfunction for patients of MMD in near future.

Suggested Readings

[1] Amarenco P, Bogousslavsky J, Caplan LR, Donnan GA, Wolf ME, Hennerici MG. The ASCOD phenotyping of ischemic stroke (Updated ASCO Phenotyping). Cerebrovasc Dis. 2013; 36(1):1–5

[2] Fukuoka S, Suematsu K, Nakamura J, Matsuzaki T, Satoh S, Hashimoto I. Transient ischemic attacks caused by unruptured intracranial aneurysms. Surg Neurol. 1982; 17(6):464–467

[3] Hernesniemi JA, Dashti R, Juvela S, Väärt K, Niemelä M, Laakso A. Natural history of brain arteriovenous malformations: a long-term follow-up study of risk of hemorrhage in 238 patients. Neurosurgery. 2008; 63(5):823–829, discussion 829–831

[4] Goehre F, Kamiyama H, Kosaka A, et al. The anterior temporal approach for microsurgical thromboembolectomy of an acute proximal posterior cerebral artery occlusion. Neurosurgery. 2014; 10(2) Suppl 2:174–178, 178

[5] Goehre F, Yanagisawa T, Kamiyama H, et al. Direct Microsurgical Embolectomy for an Acute Distal Basilar Artery Occlusion. World Neurosurg. 2016; 86:497–502

[6] Hart RG, Diener HC, Coutts SB, et al. Cryptogenic Stroke/ESUS International Working Group. Embolic strokes of undetermined source: the case for a new clinical construct. Lancet Neurol. 2014; 13(4):429–438

[7] Jeon JP, Kim JE, Cho WS, Bang JS, Son YJ, Oh CW. Meta-analysis of the surgical outcomes of symptomatic moyamoya disease in adults. J Neurosurg. 2017; •••:1–7

[8] Kazumata K, Tha KK, Narita H, et al. Chronic ischemia alters brain microstructural integrity and cognitive performance in adult moyamoya disease. Stroke. 2015; 46(2):354–360

[9] Kuroda S, Houkin K. Moyamoya disease: current concepts and future perspectives. Lancet Neurol. 2008; 7(11):1056–1066

[10] Lee KC, Joo JY, Lee KS, Shin YS. Recanalization of completely thrombosed giant aneurysm: case report. Surg Neurol. 1999; 51(1):94–98

[11] Mohr JP, Parides MK, Stapf C, et al. international ARUBA investigators. Medical management with or without interventional therapy for unruptured brain arteriovenous malformations (ARUBA): a multicentre, non-blinded, randomised trial. Lancet. 2014; 383(9917):614–621

[12] Oh YS, Lee SJ, Shon YM, Yang DW, Kim BS, Cho AH. Incidental unruptured intracranial aneurysms in patients with acute ischemic stroke. Cerebrovasc Dis. 2008; 26(6):650–653

[13] Suzuki J, Takaku A. Cerebrovascular "moyamoya" disease. Disease showing abnormal net-like vessels in base of brain. Arch Neurol. 1969; 20(3):288–299

[14] Research Committee on the Pathology and Treatment of Spontaneous Occlusion of the Circle of Willis, Health Labour Sciences Research Grant for Research on Measures for Infractable Diseases. Guidelines for diagnosis and treatment of moyamoya disease (spontaneous occlusion of the circle of Willis). Neurol Med Chir (Tokyo). 2012; 52(5):245–266

[15] Rannikmäe K, Woodfield R, Anderson CS, et al. Reliability of intracerebral hemorrhage classification systems: A systematic review. Int J Stroke. 2016; 11(6):626–636

[16] Yang MH, Lin HY, Fu J, Roodrajeetsing G, Shi SL, Xiao SW. Decompressive hemicraniectomy in patients with malignant middle cerebral artery infarction: A systematic review and meta-analysis. Surgeon. 2015; 13(4):230–240

[17] Ziai WC, Tuhrim S, Lane K, et al. CLEAR III Investigators. A multicenter, randomized, double-blinded, placebo-controlled phase III study of Clot Lysis Evaluation of Accelerated Resolu-tion of Intraventricular Hemorrhage (CLEAR III). Int J Stroke. 2014; 9(4):536–542

[18] Qureshi AI, Mohammad Y, Yahia AM, et al. Ischemic events associated with unruptured intracranial aneur-ysms: multicenter clinical study and review of the litera-ture. Neurosurgery. 2000; 46(2):282–289, discussion 289–290

6 Endovascular Intervention in the Management of Ischemic Stroke: Scientific Evidence

Adam A. Dmytriw and Vitor M. Pereira

Abstract

After being staggered by numerous negative trials in 2013, the interventional stroke community saw four years of vindication for mechanical thrombectomy showing efficacy and safety, even beyond a hopeful 6-8 hour window out to 24 h. A landmark set of five trials in 2015 provided a foundation upon which years of incremental follow-ups, meta-analyses and new breakthroughs would be built. With optimized devices for thrombectomy and image analysis, the neurointerventional community has turned to workflow and systemization in this new era of acute ischemic stroke treatment. The aim of this review is to chronicle the evidence in the epoch of positive trials, synthesize ancillary studies to these, and discuss the imminent challenges that remain.

Keywords: ischemic, stroke, neuroradiology, endovascular, reperfusion, trials

6.1 Three Strikes & Striking Out on a New Path

In 2013, three major randomized controlled trials (RCTs) comparing the effectiveness of endovascular approaches to intravenous (IV) tissue plasminogen activator (tPA) for acute stroke were published—the Interventional Management of Stroke (IMS) III, Local Versus Systemic Thrombolysis for Acute Ischemic Stroke (SYNTHESIS), and Mechanical Retrieval and Recanalization of Stroke Clots Using Embolectomy (MR RESCUE)—all of which showed negative results. However, the neurointerventional community has reason strongly to feel that these RCTs were not representative of the contemporary mechanical thrombectomy landscape. Common criticisms included marked heterogeneity in use of modern stent retrievers, delays in treatment time, and lack of baseline imaging. As such, new trials were conceived which pitted contemporary stent retrievers against medical standard care, this time with a focus of reducing door-to-puncture times and ensuring baseline computed tomography angiography (CTA) was performed.

Learning from the lessons of the three major strikes against stroke intervention (i.e., IMS III, SYNTHESIS and MR RESCUE), a new era debuted with MR CLEAN, ESCAPE, EXTEND IA, SWIFT PRIME and REVASCAT, THRACE and THERAPY. Excepting THERAPY, which was underpowered at the time of its termination, these trials would come to be known as heralds of the new epoch of positive evidence of mechanical therapy.

The first of these trials was directed in the Netherlands and was called MR CLEAN. The trail enrolled 233 participants presenting with emergent large vessel occlusion (ELVO) of the anterior circulation (intracranial internal carotid artery [ICA] and promixal middle cerebral artery [MCA]) who were randomized to endovascular treatments with usual care, while another 267 were randomized to standard of care. Ultimately, 196 underwent endovascular treatment, and 190 were treated with modern stent retrievers. Occlusion was always confirmed via CTA, and patients were treated within 6 hours of ictus with an NIHSS of ≥ 2. As is now famous, there were significant differences between patients who achieved a good functional outcome (Modified Ranking Scale [mRS] ≤ 2) in the endovascular arm (32.6%) and the standard of care arm (19.1%), with an adjusted odds ratio of 1.67 (95% CI 1.21 to 2.30). There were no significant differences in mortality, rate of symptomatic intracerebral hemorrhage (sICH), or other serious adverse events. It is now accepted that the remarkable result of MR CLEAN relative to the three negative trials is owed to a standard of baseline imaging and modern stent retrievers. Importantly, most patients were included after they had failed to respond to 1 hour of IV tPA. Thus it was known in these patients that standard of care was approaching futility. At the time of the study, the Dutch health system only permitted endovascular therapy in the context of the trial, reducing selection bias in favor of easier patients. MR CLEAN possessed the longest onset to puncture (~260 minutes) of any of the modern trials.

The culmination of MR CLEAN caused pandemonium within the endovascular community, and spurred investigators across the world to urgently perform interim analysis of their data. The ESCAPE trial was the first of these to do so and discovered a result in favor of mechanical thrombectomy which mandated cessation of the trial on safety grounds. This international trial randomized 165 patients to the endovascular plus standard care arm and 150 to the standard care arm, albeit with a timeline extended to 12 hours post ictus. Furthermore, small infarct cores were one of the explicit inclusion criteria, as well as the presence of moderate-to-good collateral circulation as identified on computed tomography perfusion (CTP) and CTA. Within the endovascular group, the incidence of functional independence (mRS ≤ 2) at 90 days (53.0% vs. 29.3%) was significantly greater, with a common odds ration (OR) of 2.6. Moreover, the number needed to treat (NNT) was onlyfour, which was stunning, as it had already dwarfed the efficacy of primary percutaneous coronary intervention. There was also an overall reduction in mortality (10.4% vs. 19%) in favor of intervention, with no difference in sICH. While MR CLEAN and ESCAPE are certainly akin, the differences are felt to be attributable to a mean time from ictus to puncture of 185 minutes and the exclusion of large infarct cores as well as poor collaterals. General anesthesia was also less commonly employed.

▶ Table 6.1

6.2 The Solitary Armamentarium

Following the heartening results emanating from Rotterdam and Calgary, EXTEND IA, SWIFTPRIME, and REVASCAT sought specifically to compare the Solitaire stent retriever (Medtronic), rather than the comparatively heterogeneous trials which permitted also the use of Trevo (Stryker) devices among others. Conducted in Australia and New Zealand, EXTEND IA randomized patients receiving IV tPA within 4.5 hours of ictus to additional Solitaire thombectomy. Seeking to further optimize imaging selection in patients, RAPID CTP software was employed identify ischemic penumbra in a standardized fashion. Whilst the study planned to enroll 100 patients with occlusions of the ICA or MCA, the results were so overwhelmingly positive at 35 patients that the trial was ceased. In addition, coprimary outcomes of 24-hour MRI reperfusion and 3-day NIHSS both overwhelmingly supported mechanical thrombectomy, with 100% reperfusion of the ischemic territory with Solitaire (37% with IV thrombolysis). Furthermore, a ≥ 8-point reduction on the NIHSS, or a score of 0 or 1, was achieved in 80% of thrombec-

tomy patients (again 36% with thrombolysis). Good functional outcome at 90 days was 71% vs. 40%, with no significant difference in rates of sICH or mortality. Here, ictus to puncture averaged 210 minutes, and rates of vascularization (86%) were the highest ever.

Conducted in the United States, Canada, and Europe, SWIFT PRIME limited its inclusion to 6 hours post ictus and the Solitaire device. Devised to randomize 477 patients between standard treatment and Solitaire with intracranial ICA, M1 or carotid terminus occlusions and absence of large ischemic core lesions on CTA or MRA, it was halted due to efficacy at ad hoc analysis of 196 patients. Using the usual good outcome measures of mRS ≤ 2 and disability at 90 days, the endovascular NNT was 2.6, functional independence was achieved in 60% (vs. 35%) with no differences in mortality and sICH rates. Here, ictus-to-puncture time averaged 224 minutes. Taking stock of the functional independences achieved at the time, the neurointerventional community noted that this was higher than MR CLEAN and emphasized efficiency and speed of workflow. In ascending order of functional independence, the trials stood at: MR CLEAN, 33%; ESCAPE, 53%; SWIFT PRIME, 60%; and EXTEND IA, 71%. (▶ Table 6.2).

6.3 Variations & Hope for the Contraindicated

In the trials to follow, provocative data would emerge regarding patients ineligible for tPA, those with larger infarct cores and poor non-contrast-enhanced CT (NECT) findings among others.

Next to completion was the trial operated out of Spain entitled REVASCAT, remarkable for its study population of those who were refractory or contraindicated to IV tPA with confirmed proximal anterior circulation occlusion. Patients were excluded by Alberta Stroke Program Early Computer Tomography Score (ASPECTS) on noncontrast CT or diffusion-weighted MRI as a surrogate for large infarct core. Another Solitaire-only trial, it was prematurely halted at 206 enrolled patients for overwhelming evidence of reduction in disability as defined by mRS with an OR for 1-point improvement on the mRS scale of 1.7 (95% CI 1.05–2.8). Once again, a rates of functional independence (mRS ≤ 2) at 90 days favored thrombectomy at 43.7% (28.2% for thrombolysis alone). Here, the NNT to prevent functional dependence was 6.5, and the sICH and mortality rates as ever were not

Table 6.1 Designs of the major

	Arms	Size	Era	Centers	Age range	Clinical criteria	Vessel occlusion	Time sindow (onset to groin puncture)	CT criteria	Advanced imaging criteria
MR RESCUE	Rescue MT vs. standard	118	2004–2011	North America (22 sites)	18–85	NIHSS 6–29	CTA/MRA showing persistent occlusion post IVT (ICA, M1, or M2)	<8 h	None	Penumbra assessment with multimodal CT or MRI only for stratification
IMS III	Bridging (various) vs. IVT	656	Aug 2006–Apr 2012	58 Centers (United States, Canada, Australia, Europe)	18–82	NIHSS ≥10 or NIHSS 8–9 with proven vessel occlusion	Not required at randomization	<5 h	None	ICA, M1, BA for proven occlusion
SYNTHESIS	MT vs. IVT	362 (181 vs. 181)	Feb 2008-Apr 2012	Italy (24 centers)	18–80	NIHSS >25 excluded	Not required at randomization	<4.5 h	None	None
THERAPY	Bridging (various) vs. IVT	108 (55 vs. 53)	Mar 2012-Oct 2014	36 Centers (United States and Germany)	18–85	NIHSS ≥8	I-ICA, M1	eligible for tPA (<4.5 h)	Excluded ischemic changes >1/3 MCA	Clot length ≥8 mm
MR CLEAN	MT vs. standard	500 (233 vs. 267)	Dec 2010-Mar 2014	Netherlands - 16 centers	≥18	NIHSS ≥2	I-ICA,M1,M2,A1,A2 *Extracranial ICA/dissection discretional*	<6 h	None	None
ESCAPE	MT vs. standard	315 (165 vs. 150)	Feb 2013-Oct 2014	22 Centers (Canada, United States, Ireland, South Korea, UK)	≥18	NIHSS >5	I-ICA,M1, 2-M2s, A1 *Extracranial ICA/dissection discretional*	<12 h	ASPECTS >5	CTA filling >50% of MCA pial collaterals, CTP = vICBF/CBV ASPECTS >5

Table 6.1 (continued)

	Arms	Size	Era	Centers	Age range	Clinical criteria	Vessel occlusion	Time sindow (onset to groin puncture)	CT criteria	Advanced imaging criteria
EXTEND IA	Bridging (Solitaire) vs. IVT	75 (35 vs. 35)	Aug 2012-Oct 2014	10 centers (9 Australia, 1 New Zealand)	≥18	No NIHSS cutoff	ICA, M1 or M2 dissection excluded	<6 h	None	Target mismatch: mismatch>1.2, rCBF core<70ml, 6 sec Tmax penumbra>10ml
SWIFT PRIME	Bridging (Solitaire) vs. IVT	196 (98 vs. 98)	Dec 2012-Nov 2014	39 centers (United States and Europe)	18–80	NIHSS 8–29	I-ICA, M1 Extra-cranial-ICA excluded (including dissection)	<6 h	Revised small core (ASPECTS >5)	Initially target mismatch (core<50ml, 10 sec Tmax lesion<100ml, penumbra >15ml and mismatch ≥1.8)
REVASCAT	MT (Solitaire) vs. standard	206 (103 vs. 103)	Nov 2012-Dec 2014	4 centers (Spain)	18–80	NIHSS>5	I-ICA, M1,	<8 h	ASPECTS>6 (>5 on DWI)	No recanalization on CTA/MRA after ≥30 tPA infusion If CTA/MRA performed >4.5 hr from onset then CBV ASPECTS, CTA-SI ASPECTS or DWI-MR ASPECTS
THRACE	Bridging vs. IVT	412 (208 vs. 204)	June 2010-Feb 2015	26 centers (France [Mothership only modell])	18–80	NIHSS 10–25	I-ICA, M1, upper one-third basilar artery, Ipsilateral E-ICA, stenosis/occlusion excluded	<5 h	None	None

Table 6.2 Major trial baseline characteristics

	Age (median)	Male (%)	NIHSS (median)	Vessel occlusion	Tandem lesion (extrancranial ICA occlusion)	ASPECTS (median)	IVT (%)	Retrievable stent (%)
MR RESCUE	66	50	16	71% ICA or M1	unreported	predicted core 36 ml	47	0
IMS III	69	50	17	18% of EVT group had no occlusion	unreported	unreported	100	4
SYNTHESIS	66	59	13	2% no occlusion	unreported	unreported	0	41
THERAPY	67	62	17	89% I-ICA or M1	excluded	7.5	100	13% (majority used aspiration thrombectomy)
MR CLEAN	66	58	17	92% I-ICA, carotid T or M1	32%	9	87 (44% drip and ship)	82
ESCAPE	71	48 (87% white)	16	96% carotid T/L or M1	13%	9	73	73
EXTEND_IA	69	49	17	88% I-ICA or M1	n/r	n/r (median core 12 ml)	100	100
SWIFT PRIME	65	55 (89% white)	17	86% carotid T/L or M1	excluded	9	100 (44% drip and ship)	100
REVASCAT	65	55	17	90% carotid T/L or M1		7	70	70
THRACE	66	57	18	98% ICA or M1	excluded	unreported	100 (100% mothership)	77

significantly different. Notably, the trial was akin to MR CLEAN in its exclusion of early response to IV tPA, unlike the other trials. Arguably, this more accurately reflected practice at the time and was an appealing aspect of the investigation. However, this by definition implied longer door-to-puncture times, and lower rates of reperfusion were unsurprising. Also, given that ASPECTS governed selection alone, larger infarct cores were present, arguably another reality of stroke intervention at the time.

Following what is now described as the five major trials of 2015 in the canon of stroke intervention, THRACE and THERAPY provided new evidence the following year. Operating out of France, THRACE compared IV tPA alone with IV tPA plus mechanical thrombectomy in a manner similar to MR CLEAN and ESCAPE. While stent retrievers were commonly the tool of choice, aspiration was permitted. Although the intent was to include CTA or MRA-confirmed ELVOs, occlusion of the superior basilar artery was also included. However, only two such patients were ultimately enrolled. With THRACE, the mandates were thrombolysis within 4 hours and thrombectomy within 5 hours of ictus. Just as with their peers, an unscheduled analysis was carried out after the (itself unplanned) conclusion of ESCAPE. Here, 208 patients were randomized to receive tPA alone, while 204 patients were to receive tPA plus mechanical thrombectomy.Functional independence (mRS ≤ 2) at 90 days favored thrombectomy at 53% (OR=1.55, 95% CI 1.05–2.30) compared to 42% with tPA alone.

Notable differences with THRACE included the fact that 30% of patients who scored 0–4 on ASPECTS nevertheless achieved functional independence at 90 days, the first glimmer that perhaps the patient with poor outlook on NECT should not be passed by. In a similar vein, investigators did not wait for response to tPA to initiate thrombectomy. As a direct consequence, 30% crossover occurred from mechanical thrombectomy to control. These factors expectedly yielded a more tempered absolute difference in functional independence compared with its contemporaries, and yet the efficacy of mechanical thrombectomy without exclusion of patients with large ischemic cores and an initial response to IV tPA was nevertheless incontrovertible. (▶ Table 6.3).

6.4 Great Aspirations, New Adaptations

Contemporaneously, the German-American study THERAPY was also terminated due to equipoise at 109 patients of a planned 692. Utilizing largely the same paradigms as their forebears, the trial differed in that the endovascular modality was exclusively that of the Penumbra aspiration system. Another distinctive criterion was the permission of ELVA with thrombus length ≥ 8 mm. The data favored intervention over control (OR=1.76, 95% CI 0.86–3.59), however the study was underpowered, and assessment of functional independence could not be adequately assessed. THERAPY was the first study to examine the effect of aspiration devices alone but did not have the power to suggest by itself whether there was a meaningful difference between stent retriever or aspiration technique.

One of the most contemporary advances in suction thrombectomy is a direct aspiration first pass technique (ADAPT), combining a large-bore catheter with a stent retriever, where the large-bore catheter is first passed to remove the clot via aspiration. While a stent retriever can be inserted afterwards for a second attempt as necessary, the technique is nevertheless inexpensive and has been shown not to significantly increase procedure time. While no randomized trial has addressed this topic, a systematic review from Australia pooled the results from 17 studies on the ADAPT technique and six RCTs on stent retrievers (IMS III, ESCAPE, EXTEND, MR CLEAN, REVASCAT, and SWIFT PRIME). The pooled results favored ADAPT technique over stent retrievers (89.6% vs. 67.2%, p < 0.001), but functional outcome (mRS ≤ 2 at 90 days) was not statistically different between the two groups. The secondary outcome of excellent functional outcome (mRS ≤ 1) at 90 days favored ADAPT but only trended towards significance. sICH and mortality rates did not significantly differ. Time from symptom onset to groin puncture was lower in the ADAPT group, but this also failed to reach significance, and this has since been confirmed by several retrospective studies. Though higher recanalization rates were observed, there were no differences detected in the functional outcomes. Nevertheless, it is often currently held that aspiration should be attempted first. (▶ Table 6.4).

Table 6.3 Individual process times

	Onset to IVT (median, min)	Onset to randomization (median, min)	Onset to groin puncture (median, min)	Onset to first reperfusion (median, min)	Groin puncture to reperfusion (median, min)	IVT to groin puncture (median, min)	CT to groin puncture (median, min)	CT to reperfusion (median, min)
MR RESCUE	unreported	unreported	381	unreported	unreported	unreported	124	unreported
IMS III	122	unreported	208	unreported	unreported	unreported	unreported	unreported
SYNTHESIS	165	148	225	unreported	unreported	unreported	unreported	unreported
THERAPY	108	181	227	unreported	unreported	unreported	123	unreported
MR CLEAN	85	204	260	332	unreported	unreported	unreported	unreported
ESCAPE	110	169	208	241	30	51	51	84
EXTEND_IA	127	256	210	248	43	74	93	unreported
SWIFT PRIME	111	191	244	252	unreported	unreported	58	87
REVASCAT	118	223	269	355	59	unreported	67	unreported
THRACE	150	168	250	unreported	unreported	unreported	unreported	unreported

6.5 Post-Hoc Perspectives

After publication of these landmark trials, it became clear that as they streamlined workflow to reduce door-to-treatment times and employed innovating imaging techniques for optimal patient selection, these new trials had unmasked remarkable benefit in functional outcomes, neurological improvement, reperfusion rates, and even mortality. The NNT to prevent one functional disability was staggeringly low, ranging from 4–6.5. In order to make the jump from remarkable to indubitable, four meta-analyses were published in 2015 and 2016.

The first of these to press hailed from Toronto and was published in *the Journal of the American Medical Association*. Comprising eight RCTs (IMS III, SYNTHESIS, MR RESCUE, MR CLEAN, ESCAPE, EXTEND-IA, SWIFT-PRIME, and REVASCAT) and a total of 2,423 patients (1,313 endovascular therapy and 1,110 standard), the OR of an improved mRS was shown to be 1.56 (95% CI 1.14–2.13). The OR for functional independence (mRS ≤ 2) at 90 days was 1.71 (95% CI 1.18–2.49), 12% greater than standard of care. As is now considered unsurprising, the OR for revascularization was 6.49 (95% CI 4.79–8.79), with 75.8% of endovascular and 34.1% of thrombolysis patients with no differences in sICH or all-cause mortality at 90 days. Subgroup and sensitivity analyses were performed, particularly given heterogeneity for mRS, showing significantly improved functional outcomes.

The next to follow was published in *Stroke* in March 2016 and comprised patient-level data from ESCAPE, SWIFT PRIME, EXTEND-IA, and REVASCAT. The primary analysis included 787 patients (401 endovascular group and 386 standard) from these Solitaire-predominant trials. As had become quotidian, primary outcome was functional score at 90 days (by the mRS) and secondary outcomes were functional independence (mRS ≤ 2), mortality and sICH rates. The *Stroke* meta-analysis showed a common odds ratio (cOR) for mRS improvement of 2.7 (95% CI 2.0–3.5), with NNTs of 2.5 and 4.25 to reduce disability and for better functional outcome, respectively. Mortality and sICH rates did not differ meaningfully. Moreover, there were two sensitivity analyses in which ESCAPE was excluded, as well as a separate analysis for any other non-Solitaire usage, with similar results to the primary analysis. The benefit of thrombectomy was consistently observed across all subgroups, including age, sex, NIHSS score, site of lesion, presence of tandem occlusions, and ASPECTS. Impor-

Table 6.4 Major trial outcomes by era

	Recanalization (%, EVT vs. control)	Reperfusion (mTICI 2b/3, %)	Primary outcome	mRS at day 90	mRS 0–2 at day 90	Final infarct volume (mL)	sICH (PH-2, %)	Death at day 90 (%)	New AIS in a different territory (%)	SAE (%)
MR RESCUE	69	27	mRS 3.8 vs. 3.4	3.8 vs. 3.4	21 vs. 26	32 vs. 32	9 vs. 6	18 vs. 21	1.4	62
IMS III	81 ICA; 86 M1; 88 M2	38 ICA; 44 M1; 44 M2	mRS 0–2 41 vs. 39%	nr	41 vs. 39	nr	6 vs. 6	19 vs. 21	nr	nr
SYNTHESIS	nr	nr	mRS 0–1 30 vs. 35%	nr	42 vs. 46	nr	6 vs. 6	8 vs. 6	nr	nr
PISTE	69	87	OR 2.12 mRS 0–2 p = 0.2	nr	51 vs. 40 vs NNT = 9	nr	0 vs. 0	7 vs. 4	nr	45 vs. 34
THERAPY	nr	70	mRS 0–2 38 vs. 30% p = 0.44	nr	38 vs. 30 ns	nr	9.3 vs. 9.7	12 vs. 24	nr	42 vs. 48
MR CLEAN	75 v 33	59	mRS 3 v. 4 day 90	3 vs. 4	33 vs. 19 NNT = 7	49 vs. 79	6 vs. 5	21 vs. 22	5.6	47 vs. 42
ESCAPE	nr vs. 31 (mAOL 2–3)	72	cOR 2.6	2 vs. 4	53 vs. 29 NNT = 4	nr	4 vs. 3	10 vs. 19 (significant)	nr	21 vs. 18
EXTEND_IA	94 vs. 43 (TIMI 2–3)	86	24-h reperfusion 100 vs. 37% Early neurological recovery 82 vs. 37%	1 v 3	71 vs. 40 NNT = 3	23 vs. 53	0 vs. 6	9 vs. 20 (p = 0.18)	5.7	nr
SWIFT PRIME	nr	88	Shift analysis p = 0.0002	2 vs. 3	60 vs. 36 NNT = 4	nr	1 vs. 3	9 vs. 12 (p = 0.5)	nr	36 vs. 31
REVASCAT	nr	66	cOR 1.7	nr	44 vs. 28 NNT = 6	16 vs. 39	5 vs. 2	18 vs. 16	5	30 vs. 25
THRACE	78	69	mRS 0–2 at day 90 53% v. 42%	nr	53 v. 42 NNT = 9	nr	2 vs. 2	12 vs. 13	6	8 vs. 7

tantly, the meta-analysis suggested there is no evidence of reduced benefit in the elderly (≥ 80 years of age), and in fact there was an observed clinically significant 20% absolute reduction in mortality rates. This was extraordinarily meaningful for this population, in whom thrombolysis is usually contraindicated. Another subgroup was NIHSS, as both IMS III and MR CLEAN partly selected patients of this basis. However, there was no significant difference in benefit between NIHSS ≤ 15 and NIHSS > 20 patients. Unsurprisingly, pooled data affirmed better functional outcome with lower time from onset to intervention.

Incorporating a greater number of trials, a Portuguese study published in *The BMJ* included all 2,925 from IMS III, SYNTHESIS, MR RESCUE, MR CLEAN, ESCAPE, EXTEND-IA, SWIFT-PRIME, REVASCAT, THERAPY, and THRACE. These pooled data showed a a risk ratio of 1.37 (95% CI 1.14–1.64) for good functional outcome (mRS ≤ 2) with no significant difference in mortality or sICH. The authors conceded that the heterogeneity of the studies was high. They ameliorated this with exclusion of MR RESCUE, SYNTHESIS, and IMS III (i.e., the 2013 trials), such that the RR improved to 1.56 (95% CI 1.38 to 1.75), which was felt to be a more faithful reflection of current practice outcomes.

Lastly, the Highly Effective Reperfusion Evaluated in Multiple Endovascular Stroke Trials (HERMES) meta analysis published in the Lancet concentrated on the five breakout 2015 trials, namely, MR CLEAN, ESCAPE, EXTEND-IA, SWIFT-PRIME, and REVASCAT. Comprising 1,287 patients (634 endovascular group and 653 standard). These pooled results offered an adjusted cOR of 2.49 (95% CI 1.76–3.53) in favor of thrombectomy for significant reduction of disability (mRS at 90 days), with an NNT of 2.6 to reduce mRS by one point or greater. Once again as regards subgroups, patients > 80 years of age achieved a cOR of 3.68 (95% CI 1.95–6.92), and patients who were randomized 300 minutes post ictus achieved a cOR of 1.79 (95% CI 1.05–2.97). In addition, thrombolysis ineligible patients had cOR of 2.43 (95% CI 1.30–4.55), completing the troika of heartening data in these poor-prognosis populations.

While these meta-analyses are compelling in their pooling of the new age trials, they were also remarkable in that functional outcome was better even with the inclusion of the negative three-strikes trials. Beyond this, there was the undeniably-provocative suggestion that thrombolysis is effective regardless of patient age, NIHSS score,

ASPECTS score, site of lesion, presence of tandem cervical carotid occlusions, delay in randomization, or potentially even presence of tPA. With these analyses in hand, the neurointerventional community was armed with a compelling argument to emphasize building health care systems that increase the presence of and access to comprehensive stroke centers.

6.6 Thrombolysis, Tandems, and Therapeutic Sedation

A much-debated area of concern is the advantage or lack thereof concerning thrombolysis in patients who are considered for mechanical thrombectomy. Commonly-described benefits of thrombolysis include potential for early recanalization, clot mollification prior to intervention, and bailout in the setting of thrombectomy failure. Importantly though rate was the case then thrombolysis was response was early. Conversely, tPA is a potent drug replete with risks, including theoretical increase in sICH, clot fragmentation, and distal embolization, as well as potential delay in thrombectomy. In a post hoc analysis of data from the Solitaire Flow Restoration Thrombectomy for Acute Revascularization (STAR) and SWIFT trials, MT with IV tPA was compared with MT alone. Out of 291 patients available for analysis, 131 received only MT and 160 received both IV tPA and MT. There were no statistically significant differences found in any outcome, including time from symptom onset to groin puncture, number of passes required, rate of successful reperfusion, functional independence (mRS ≤ 2) at 90 days, mortality at 90 days, risk of emboli to new territory, sICH rates, and vasospasm.

A meta-analysis performed out of Australia and the United States looked at 12 comparative studies comprising 1,275 endovascular-only and 1,340 endovascular plus tPA patients. Naturally, the investigators found a greater proportion of coronary artery disease (CAD), transient ischemic attack (TIA)m and atrial fibrillation (aFib) in the endovascular-only arm. Nevertheless, there were no differences in procedure time, the modified thrombolysis in cerebral infarction grade, or sICH. Moreover, differences in good functional outcomes at 90 days (mRS ≤ 2) were not significant. Mortality and functional outcome were similar.

The same group proceeded to then perform a Bayesian network meta-analysis in cooperation with Canada and the United Kingdom, not only comparing as distinct groups patients with and without thrombolysis before MT, but also separating out those who underwent MT and were contraindicated to tPA. It compared 3,161 patients (five RCTs and seven prospective cohort studies), which in addition to establishing findings of no significant difference in outcome between treatment groups also clarified that there was no difference in mortality and further revealed higher rates of reperfusion without tPA. Ahead of an RCT on the subject, the authors concluded with the provocative statement that thrombolysis may not be associated with improved outcomes.

Secondly, the incidence of tandem occlusion is reported to be in the range of 20% (17% in ESCAPE, 32.3% in MR CLEAN, 18.6% in REVASCAT) and the rate of recanalization for carotid occlusion or near-occlusion with systemic thrombolysis is in the range of 9% with tandem ICA and MCA occlusions. Moreover, in the setting of tandem occlusion, there is currently no consensus on whether conservative management using mechanical thrombectomy only or some variant of more aggressive management employing angioplasty with or without stenting should be preferred. Importantly, however, the treatment was found to be safe in the two major trials which permitted its management. In addition, case time was comparable with patients who did not have extracranial intervention. A recent meta-analysis conducted in Italy corroborates this, except with same-session stenting.

The order of operations is also contested. When the extracranial occlusion is impassable with a catheter, the dilemma is removed. When not mandatory to address this, arguments in favor include improving the opportunity for collateral flow and access to the clot, as well as ease of withdrawal. Proponents of the reverse operation invoke the maxim of "time is brain" and a theoretical risk of increased complications and distal embolization. Relatedly, there is considerable debate about when a stent should be placed in concert with angioplasty. This is currently discretional, usually dependent on the degree of stenosis remaining. Of paramount concern is superimposing antiplatelet agents to prevent in-stent thrombosis with systemic thrombolysis, with small studies showing increased sICH. This scenario offers yet another situation in which there may be cause to forego thrombolysis. Complicating this further is the fact that CTA often underestimates dissection, as the gantry often outpaces slow-moving contrast boluses.

Another controversy which remains in the current era is the choice between general anesthesia with intubation and neuroleptanesthsia (conscious sedation). The cited advantages of general anesthesia include involving less pain, anxiety, patient movement, and aspiration risk. Neuroleptanesthsia is less time-consuming, theoretically affords provides more hemodynamic stability, avoids risks associated with intubation and induction, and permits real-time neurological status assessment. Chief among these concerns is the induction phase, where transient hypotension is feared to deprive a substrate which is already hypoperfused.

The first large-scale evidence arose from a meta-analysis which showed an OR of 2.59 (CI, 1.87–3.58) for mortality in patients undergoing general anesthesia as well as an OR of 2.09 (% CI, 1.36–3.23) for respiratory complications and OR 0.43 (CI, 0.35– 0.53) in addition to poorer reperfusion rates. Yet another meta-analysis focusing on data from the seminal five 2015 RCTs suggested that functional outcomes were better with conscious sedation (OR, 2.08; 95% CI, 1.47–2.96).

Ultimately, a German single-center RCT Sedation vs. Intubation for Endovascular Stroke Treatment (SIESTA) conducted in 2016 randomized 150 MT patients (73 general anesthesia, 77 conscious sedation). The results came as a surprise to the majority of the neurointerventional community at the time. First, the primary outcome of neurological improvement after 24 hours (based on NIHSS) showed no significant difference. Moreover, general anesthesia was associated with better functional outcome (37.0% vs. 18.2%, P = .01). Notwithstanding associated intubation-related complications such as hypothermia, delayed extubation, and pneumonia, no difference in mortality was noted. No secondary outcomes reached significance, though functional independence approached significance in favor of general anesthesia. Reflecting on these results, it is felt that patients prior to the RCT indicated for general anesthesia commonly had more severe strokes with higher NIHSS scores. Nevertheless, this area remains hotly disputed, and the HERMES collaborators would soon return with a new meta-analysis which in fact strongly favored neuroleptanaesthesia.

6.7 Expanding the Window and the Tools

Despite having revolutionized the care of ELVO in the short span of two years from 2015–2017, the neurovascular community was not to rest on its laurels. The page had barely been turned on HERMES when on the first week of 2018, the

DAWN trial was published. This groundbreaking effort would show that when ELVO patients had last been seen well 6 to 24 hours earlier and also had a mismatch between clinical deficit and infarct volume, outcomes for disability at 90 days favored thrombectomy with an adjusted difference of 2.0 points (95% CI, 1.1 to 3.0; posterior probability of superiority, >0.999). The coprimary endpoint of the rate of functional independence at 90 days was 49% in the thrombectomy group and 13% in the control. Even with this expanded window, the rates of morality and sICH wer not significantly different. This study was also notable as the tool of the trade was changed to exclusively feature the Trevo stent retriever.

One month later, the North American study DEFUSE-3 was prematurely terminated for equipoise, and showed that MT for ELVO in patients last seen well 6 to 16 hours earlier resulted in improved outcomes as long as the at-risk region had not already infarcted. Patients were eligible if the initial infarct volume measured less than 70 mL on RAPID CTP. Here, the OR was 2.77 (95% confidence interval [CI], 1.63 to 4.70; P < 0.001) For disability scores as determined by mRS at 90 days, the risk ratio was 2.67 (95% CI, 1.60 to 4.48; P < 0.001) for functional independence. The uniform use of RAPID software is one of the hallmarks of this trial, whereas DAWN utilized diffusion-weighted imaging or CTA/CTP of any kind. Debate is ongoing regarding the utility of MRI for selection, for while it is sensitive, the DWI-ASPECTS and DWI-fluid attenuated inversion recovery studies to-date have shown suboptimal inter-rater agreement.

6.8 The Next Epochs

Rebounding from the three strikes against stroke intervention in 2013, the ensuing four years saw the effectiveness and safety of mechanical thrombectomy go from strongly suspected to incontrovertible, from well beyond the expected 6 to 8 hour window. The seminal five trials provide a foundation upon which the 2016 follow-ups could build with nuanced investigation and meta-analysis. Entering into the second epoch of mechanical thrombectomy, the neurointerventional community is now focused upon efficiency and workflow, with optimal ictus-to-puncture times, algorithmic CTP and volume techniques, suction thrombectomy adjuncts, and periprocedural considerations. Future investigation will undoubtedly be driven by all of the advances in neuroradiology (before, during, and after stroke), multifactorial clinical neurology, and endovascular techniques.

Suggested Readings

[1] Berkhemer OA, Fransen PSS, Beumer D, et al. MR CLEAN Investigators. A randomized trial of intraarterial treatment for acute ischemic stroke. N Engl J Med. 2015; 372(1):11–20

[2] Pierot L, Pereira VM, Cognard C, von Kummer R. Teaching Lessons by MR CLEAN. AJNR Am J Neuroradiol. 2015; 36(5): 819–821

[3] Goyal M, Demchuk AM, Menon BK, et al. ESCAPE Trial Investigators. Randomized assessment of rapid endovascular treatment of ischemic stroke. N Engl J Med. 2015; 372(11):1019–1030

[4] Campbell BCV, Mitchell PJ, Kleinig TJ, et al. EXTEND-IA Investigators. Endovascular therapy for ischemic stroke with perfusion-imaging selection. N Engl J Med. 2015; 372(11):1009–1018

[5] Saver JL, Goyal M, Bonafe A, et al. SWIFT PRIME Investigators. Stent-retriever thrombectomy after intravenous t-PA vs. t-PA alone in stroke. N Engl J Med. 2015; 372(24):2285–2295

[6] Jovin TG, Chamorro A, Cobo E, et al. REVASCAT Trial Investigators. Thrombectomy within 8 hours after symptom onset in ischemic stroke. N Engl J Med. 2015; 372(24):2296–2306

[7] Bracard S, Ducrocq X, Mas JL, et al. THRACE Investigators. Mechanical thrombectomy after intravenous alteplase versus alteplase alone after stroke (THRACE): a randomised controlled trial. Lancet Neurol. 2016; 15(11):1138–1147

[8] Badhiwala JH, Nassiri F, Alhazzani W, et al. Endovascular Thrombectomy for Acute Ischemic Stroke: A Meta-analysis. JAMA. 2015; 314(17):1832–1843

[9] Campbell BCV, Hill MD, Rubiera M, et al. Safety and Efficacy of Solitaire Stent Thrombectomy: Individual Patient Data Meta-Analysis of Randomized Trials. Stroke. 2016; 47(3): 798–806

[10] Rodrigues FB, Neves JB, Caldeira D, Ferro JM, Ferreira JJ, Costa J. Endovascular treatment versus medical care alone for ischaemic stroke: systematic review and meta-analysis. BMJ. 2016; 353(January):i1754

[11] Goyal M, Menon BK, van Zwam WH, et al. HERMES collaborators. Endovascular thrombectomy after large-vessel ischaemic stroke: a meta-analysis of individual patient data from five randomised trials. Lancet. 2016; 387(10029):1723–1731

[12] Phan K, Dmytriw AA, Maingard J, et al. Endovascular thrombectomy alone versus combined with intravenous thrombolysis. World Neurosurg. 2017; 108:850–858.e2

[13] Phan K. A. A. Dmytriw I. Teng, J. Moore, C. Griessenauer, C, Ogilvy, A. Thomas. direct aspiration first pass technique (ADAPT) versus standard endovascular therapy for acute stroke: a systematic review and meta-analysis. Neurosurgery. 2017

[14] Schönenberger S, Möhlenbruch M, Pfaff J, et al. Sedation vs. Intubation for Endovascular Stroke TreAtment (SIESTA) - a randomized monocentric trial. Int J Stroke. 2015; 10(6):969–978

[15] Campbell BCV, van Zwan WH, Goyal M, et al. Effect of general anaesthesia on functional outcome in patients with anterior circulation ischaemic stroke undergoing endovascular thrombectomy versus standard care: a meta-analysis of individual patient data from seven randomised controlled trials. Lancet Neurol. 2018; 17:47–53

[16] Nogueira RG, Jadhav AP, Haussen DC, et al. DAWN Trial Investigators. Thrombectomy 6 to 24 hours after stroke with a mismatch between deficit and infarct. N Engl J Med. 2018; 378(1):11–21

[17] Albers GW, Marks MP, Kemp S, et al. DEFUSE 3 Investigators. Thrombectomy for stroke at 6 to 16 hours with selection by perfusion imaging. N Engl J Med. 2018; 378(8):708–718

[18] Fahed R, Lecler A, Sabben C, et al. DWI-ASPECTS (Diffusion-Weighted Imaging-Alberta Stroke Program Early Computed Tomography Scores) and DWI-FLAIR (Diffusion-Weighted Imaging-Fluid Attenuated Inversion Recovery) Mismatch in Thrombectomy Candidates: An Intrarater and Interrater Agreement Study. Stroke. 2017; 117:019508

7 Mechanical Thrombectomy with Retrievable Stents

Carlos Castaño

Abstract

In this chapter we make a historical recount of the evolution of mechanical thrombectomy and describe the technique of mechanical thrombectomy with Retreivable stent.

Keywords: ischemic stroke, mechanical thrombectomy, retrievable stents, stent-retriever, endovascular recanalization, large vessel occlusion in acute stroke

7.1 Background and Brief History

In the last 21 years, the introduction and generalization of intravenous thrombolytic therapy (IVTT) of the stroke has been a clear advance that has benefited thousands of people.[1] The National Institute of Neurological Diseases and Stroke (NINDS) Genentech Intravenous (IV) tPA stroke trial established the critical importance of time to treatment and led to Food and Drug Administration (FDA) approval of IV tPA to treat acute ischemic stroke (AIS) in 1996, but within a small window of 3 hours.[1] However, in many patients (35–90%), IVTT does not achieve arterial recanalization, especially in cases of occlusion of a large cerebral vessel. For this reason, it was necessary to develop endovascular rescue procedures (ERP) as an effective therapeutic alternative to intravenous fibrinolytic treatment.

Local intra-arterial treatment began in the 1980s by administering fibrinolytic drugs directly to the thrombus through a microcatheter.[1] Basilar artery occlusion was felt to have the worst prognosis, and this drove Zeumer et al[2] to first perform basilar thrombolysis via catheter and report excellent outcomes based on historical controls.

Del Zoppo, Furlan, Higashida, and Pessin designed the Prolyse in Acute Cerebral Thromboembolism (PROACT, versions I and II) trials to demonstrate the safety, recanalization efficacy, and clinical benefit of Intraarterial (IA) r-proUK in patients with Middle Cerebral Artery (MCA) occlusion treated within 6 hours of stroke onset.[1,2,3,4]

In 1998, the PROACT study[3] described the efficacy of administering locally and through a microcatheter, r-proUK in cerebral arterial occlusion, demonstrating high rates of recanalization and improvement clinic. The conclusion of this work stated, "Intra-arterial local rpro-UK infusion was associated with superior recanalization in acute thrombotic/thrombolitic stroke compared with placebo."

In 1999, the results of the PROACT II study[4] showed "For the primary analysis, 40% of r-proUK patients and 25% of control patients had a modified Rankin score of 2 or less (P = 0,4). Mortality was 25% for the r-proUK group, and 27% for the control group. The recanalization rate was 66% for the r-proUK group, and 18% for the control group (P < .001). Intracranial hemorrhage with neurologic deterioration within 24 hours occurred in 10% of r-proUK patients and 2% of control patients (P = .06)." However, the FDA did not approve r-proUK for IA stroke therapy because of the small size and marginal significance (P=0.043) of PROACT II.[1]

Use of mechanical thrombectomy (MT) also began in the 1990s. Two UCLA inventors, Y. P. Gobin and J.P. Wensel, were involved in the design of a revolutionary device known as the Concentric Mechanical Embolus Removal in Cerebral Ischemia (MERCI) Retrieval. The MERCI Retrieval story started in the fall of 1995, when Gobin saw the need for a device that would just remove the clot and would be faster and have less risk of hemorrhage than thrombolytics. In 1996, Gobin and Wensel started in vitro studies and then animal studies. In May 2001, clinical lab safety studies began, leading to success. The first two patients treated at UCLA with the MERCI Retriever were two full Thrombolysis in Myocardial Infarction (TIMI) score 3.[5] The MERCI Retriever device received an FDA pre-market approval in 2004 and was the first device to be used for clot removal in AIS.

In 2005, the first MERCI trial was published.[6] In this trial, the recanalization was achieved in 46% (69/151) of patients with intention to treat analysis and in 48% (68/141) of patients in whom the device was deployed. This rate is significantly higher than expected, using an historical control of 18% (P 0.0001). Clinically significant procedural complications occurred in 10 of 141 (7.1%) patients. Symptomatic intracranial hemorrhages were observed in 11 of 141 (7.8%) patients. Good neurologic outcomes (modified Rankin score < 2) were more frequent at 90 days in patients with successful recanalization compared with patients with unsuccessful recanalization (46% vs. 10%; relative risk [RR], 4.4; 95% CI, 2.1 to 9.3; P = 0.0001), and mortality was less (32% vs. 54%; RR, 0.59; 95% CI, 0.39 to 0.89; P = 0.01).

In 2008, the Multi MERCI Trial was published.[7] In this trial, 164 patients received thrombectomy, and 131 were initially treated with the L5 Retriever. Mean age ± SD was 68 ± 16 years, and baseline median (interquartile range) National Institutes of Health Stroke Scale (NIHSS) score was 19 (15 to 23). Treatment with the L5 Retriever resulted in successful recanalization in 75 of 131 (57.3%) treatable vessels and in 91 of 131 (69.5%) after adjunctive therapy (IA tPA, mechanical). Overall, favorable clinical outcomes (modified Rankin Scale 0 to 2) occurred in 36%, and mortality was 34%; both outcomes were significantly related to vascular recanalization. Symptomatic intracerebral hemorrhage occurred in 16 patients (9.8%); four (2.4%) of these were parenchymal hematoma type 2. Clinically significant procedural complications occurred in nine (5.5%) patients.

In 2008 appeared the Penumbra System (Penumbra, Inc), which supposes a sophistication of the concept of thrombectomy by aspiration.[8] Initially, the technique consisted of the application of continuous aspiration by means of a suction pump simultaneously with the manipulation of the thrombus, which was carried out with a conical device that mobilized in and out of the thrombus (penumbra 3D separator), thus fragmenting it. Continuous aspiration collected these fragments and thus prevented catheter obstruction. This system was approved by the FDA in 2008 and evaluated in a first study that included 125 patients treated in less than 8 hours, of which 81.6% recanalized and 11.2% presented Symptomatic intracerebral hemorrhage (SICH), although only 25% had a good prognosis.[9] This triggered criticism about MT and the discrepancy between recanalization and prognosis. However, a subsequent study of 157 patients showed recanalization rates of 87% and mRS ≤ 2 in 41%.[10] Further technological development has seen the development of new catheters such as 5MAX, 5MAX-ACE, ACE64 and ACE68, and no longer use the 'penumbra 3D separator'. Thus, this technique has evolved a lot and is now known as A Direct Aspiration First Pass Technique (ADAPT).[11] (This technique will be developed in another chapter).

Because successful recanalization with the MERCI Retriever was achieved in less than 60% of treatable vessels (Multi MERCI trial),[7] a new device was needed that was more effective. After the MERCI Retriever came the era of stents retrievers or retrievable stents. Retrievable stents were first used for thrombectomy in 2008, when C. Castaño used the Solitaire AB stent (Medtronic), which had been designed for intracranial aneurysms[12] and had the particularity of being attached to a guide and detachable by electrolysis. Instead of detaching the stent, Castaño used it to catch the thrombus and used the guide to remove the stent with the thrombus. In June 2008, Castaño started animal studies and in November of that year treated his first patient with full TICI 3, using the Solitaire AB stent to remove the thrombus which had not been removable using the MERCI device. In 2009, he published this patient [13] in the first paper that describing technique. In August 2010, he published a pilot study with the first 20 cases.[14] In this study, successful revascularization, defined as TICI grade 2b or 3, was achieved in 18 of 20 (90%) treated vessels, and 16 patients showed immediate restoration of flow after stent deployment. The mean number of passes for maximal recanalization was 1.4, and the median (quartiles) time from groin puncture to recanalization was 50 (38–71) minutes. No case required adjuvant therapy after deployment of the embolectomy device, and no significant procedural events occurred. Symptomatic intracranial hemorrhage was found in two (10%) patients; four (20%) patients died during the 90-day follow-up period, and 45% of patients showed good functional outcome at 3 months (modified Rankin Scale score ≤ 2).

This study marked a turning point in the endovascular treatment of ischemic stroke. Subsequent studies confirmed the efficacy of the Solitaire stent for restoring vascular patency at a significantly higher rate than previous generation devices and techniques.[15,16]

In 2012, a randomized study comparing the MERCI Retriever with the Solitaire stent was published (SWIFT Trial)[15]; In this randomized, parallel-group, noninferiority trial, patients were enrolled from 18 sites (17 in the United States and one in France). Between February 2010, and February 2011, they randomly allocated 58 patients to the Solitaire group and 55 patients to the MERCI group. The primary efficacy outcome was achieved more often in the Solitaire group than in the MERCI group (61% vs. 24%; difference 37% [95% CI 19–53], odds ratio [OR] 4·87 [95% CI 2·14–11·10]; P (noninferiority) < .001, P (superiority) < .001). More patients had good 3-month neurologic outcome with Solitaire than with MERCI (58% vs. 33%;

difference 25% [6–43], OR 2.78 [1.25–6.22]; P (noninferiority) < .001, P (superiority) = 0.02). Ninety-day mortality was lower in the Solitaire group than it was in the MERCI group (17 vs. 38; difference -21% [-39 to -3], OR 0·34 [0.14–0.81]; P (noninferiority) < .001, p(superiority)=0.02).

In October 2013, a prospective, multicenter, single-arm study of MT using Solitaire Flow Restoration in AIS was published (STAR trial).[16] A total of 202 patients were enrolled across 14 comprehensive stroke centers in Europe, Canada, and Australia. The median age was 72 years; 60% were female patients. The median National Institute of Health Stroke Scale (NIHSS) was 17. Most proximal intracranial occlusion was the internal carotid artery in 18%, and the middle cerebral artery in 82%. Successful revascularization was achieved in 79.2% of patients. Device and procedure-related severe adverse events were found in 7.4%. Favorable neurologic outcome (mRS ≤ 2) was found in 57.9%. The mortality rate was 6.9%. Intracranial hemorrhagic transformation was found in 18.8% of patients; 1.5% were symptomatic.

Recently, several clinical trials (MR CLEAN,[17] EXTEND IA,[18] ESCAPE,[19] SWIFT PRIME,[20] REVAS-CAT[21])have demonstrated that thrombectomy with a retrievable stent in patients with AIS with large artery occlusion safely increases the rate of functional independence, with scientific evidence Class 1, Level A.

After these five extensive randomized studies (discussed in other chapters of this book) were published, a great number of related meta-analysis studies appeared almost simultaneously, all demonstrating the effectiveness of MT as a treatment for AIS resulting from proximal occlusion in the anterior territory.

Because proximal occlusions were so epidemiologically relevant (17–42% of AIS admissions), scientists devoted their efforts to proving that these techniques could be employed beyond the established time limits. In this way, the universe of potential patients to be rescued from this devastating disease could enlarge considerably.

Two recent trials, the long-awaited Diffusion Weighted Imaging [DWI] or Computerized Tomography Perfusion [CTP] Assessment with Clinical Mismatch in the Triage of Wake Up and Late Presenting Strokes Undergoing Neurointervention with Trevo (DAWN) trial[1], and The Endovascular Therapy Following Imaging Evaluation for Ischemic Stroke 3(DEFUSE 3),[2] have increased the time limit for endovascular treatment of AIS from 6 hours up to 24 hours in selected cases. Both trials were terminated early for efficacy due to the clear benefit for treated patients.

The DEFUSE 3 study was a multicenter, randomized, open label trial which included patients with proximal MCA or internal carotid artery (ICA) occlusion, an initial infarct size of less than 70 ml, and a ratio of ischemic tissue volume on perfusion imaging to infarct volume of 1.8 or more. One hundred eighty-two patients were randomized to medical therapy plus endovascular therapy, or medical therapy alone. The endovascular group showed better functional score at 90 days (OR, 2.77; P < 0.001) and much higher functional independence (45% vs. 17%, P < 0.001). No difference was observed for adverse effects[2].

The DAWN Trial, on the other hand, included patients with the same occlusion sites, but last seen well between 6 and 24 hours earlier, and who had a clinical mismatch between severity of the deficit and infarct volume. Two hundred six patients were enrolled and were randomized to endovascular plus standard treatment or standard treatment alone. The specified endpoint of utility-weighted modified Rankin scale at 3 months was 2 points higher in the endovascular arm (IC 95%, 1.1 to 3.0; P = > 0.999), and functional independence at 3 months or 90 days was 49% in the thrombectomy group as compared with 13% in the control group (P = > 0.999). No difference in complication rate was observed[1].

The combined findings of both trials constitute very strong evidence in favor of treatment beyond the 6-hour limit, up to 24 hours. Further evidence will be necessary to determine whether imaging mismatch evidence is necessary or can improve patient selection for the most benefit. We also believe incorporation of CTP in most centers' protocols as a standard for evaluation of AIS patients will not add significant delay and will aid in decision-making. This will be especially important in those cases in which a longer period has passed since last seen well.

7.2 Mechanical Thrombectomy Techniques

The goal of any treatment modality for AIS is to restore perfusion of ischemic tissue to improve the patient's functional prognosis. Recanalization of occlusion has been associated with improved prognosis; however, recanalization alone is not sufficient and requires the reperfusion of the cerebral parenchyma to achieve a good prognosis.[22]

In the past, many techniques were used to try to reperfusion the brain, to remove the thrombus and open the arteries, but none of them could prove its effectiveness.At present there are basically three techniques of MT in use which are showing their effectiveness:

- Proximal: Acting on the proximal part of the thrombus. This group includes the suction systems, or ADAPT, and will be discussed in another chapter.
- Distal: Once the occlusion is crossed, the force is deployed and applied to the distal parts of the thrombus, and according to the length of the device, this force is also exerted on the medial and proximal portions of the thrombus. This group includes devices with stent, brush, basket, interlinked cage forms, etc., based on the initial stent retriever (Solitaire). In this chapter we will develop this technique.

- A combination of these two, technically known as Solumbra technique.

7.3 New Devices

In recent years, multiple devices have been developed similar to the Solitaire and capable of recanalization of the cerebral arteries.

At present, the following devices are on the market:

1. Solitaire AB, Solitaire FR, Solitaire 2 (Medtronic). (▶ Fig. 7.1)
2. Trevo Retriever (Trevo ProVue Retriever, and Trevo XP ProVue Retreiver). (Stryker Neurovascular). (▶ Fig. 7.2)
3. Catch + Mechanical Thrombus Retriever (Balt Extrusion). (▶ Fig. 7.3)
4. Revive SE Thrombectomy Device (DePuySynthes). (▶ Fig. 7.4).

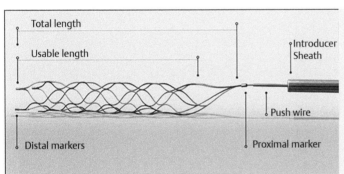

Fig. 7.1 Solitaire Retrievable Stent.

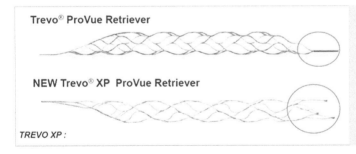

Fig. 7.2 Trevo Retriever.

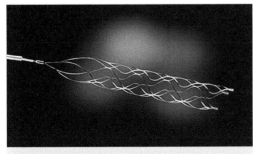

Fig. 7.3 Catch + Mechanical Thrombus Retriever.

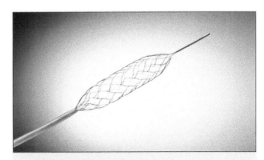

Fig. 7.4 Revive SE Thrombectomy Device.

5. APERIO Thrombectomy Device (Acandis). (► Fig. 7.5)
6. Eric Retrieval Device (Microvention). (► Fig. 7.6).

7. pREset Thrombectomy Device (Phenox). (► Fig. 7.7)
8. Phenox CRC Mechanical Thrombectomy Device (Phenox). (► Fig. 7.8)
9. EmboTrap Revascularization Device (Neuravi). (► Fig. 7.9)
10. MindFrame Capture (Medtronic). (► Fig. 7.10)
11. Golden Retriever neuro thrombectomy device (Amnis Therapeutics). (► Fig. 7.11)
12. ReStore Thrombectomy device (Medtronic). (► Fig. 7.12)

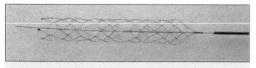

Fig. 7.5 APERIO Thrombectomy Device.

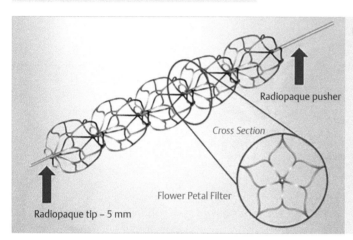

Fig. 7.6 Eric Retrieval Device.

Radiopaque pusher

Cross Section

Flower Petal Filter

Radiopaque tip – 5 mm

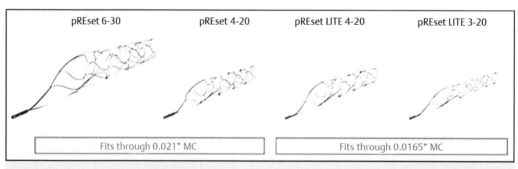

pREset 6-30   pREset 4-20   pREset LITE 4-20   pREset LITE 3-20

Fits through 0.021" MC

Fits through 0.0165" MC

Fig. 7.7 pREset Thrombectomy.

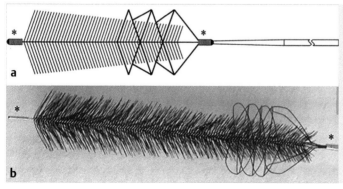

a

b

Fig. 7.8 Phenox CRC Mechanical Thrombectomy Device.

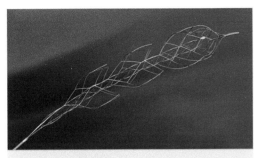

Fig. 7.9 EmboTrap Device.

7.4 Technique for Mechanical Trombectomy with Retrievable Stents (As we do in our hospital)

7.4.1 Criteria and Indications

Criteria for primary or rescue endovascular treatment were predefined and approved by the local ethics committee[23] Briefly, all patients with AIS with no contraindication for IV thrombolysis who arrived within the first 4.5 hours receive the standard dose of recombinant tissue-type plasminogen

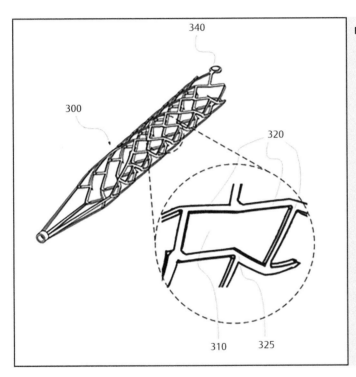

Fig. 7.10 MindFrame Capture.

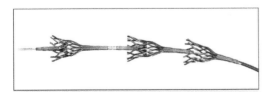

Fig. 7.11 Golden Retriever neuro thrombectomy device.

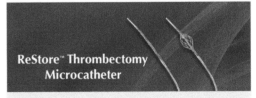

Fig. 7.12 ReStore Thrombectomy Device.

activator (0.9 mg/kg). Patients refractory to, or ineligible for, IV thrombolysis (including stroke onset more than 4.5 hours, unknown onset, or wake-up stroke) are preselected for endovascular stroke therapy according to clinical criteria (NIHSS score ≥ 6 or suspicion of large vessel occlusion) at the local centers.

Subsequently, at our comprehensive stroke center, an indication for endovascular stroke therapy is based on demonstration of a large vessel occlusion by noninvasive vascular imaging and the presence of signs of limited early infarction before transferring the patient to the angiosuite. Multimodal imaging (MRI or CT perfusion) is recommended in patients more than 4.5 hours from stroke onset.

Informed consent from the patients or their relatives is obtained before the endovascular procedure.

After the procedure, patients are admitted to an acute stroke unit and managed according to the European Stroke Organization Guidelines.[24] A CT scan is performed routinely at 24–36 hours after treatment, or earlier if any neurologic worsening ≥ 4 points in NIHSS score occurs.

7.5 Revascularization Procedure

Depending on the patient's condition, procedures are performed under sedation or general anesthesia.

Technical details of the procedure have been previously described by us.[14,25]

7.5.1 Transfemoral Approach

The standard endovascular approach to acute stroke intervention is the common femoral approach. The preference for this approach is related to the compressibility of the right common femoral artery, the potential for less dire consequences in case of femoral artery injury compared to carotid artery injury, and the fact that via this approach all brachiocephalic vessels can be catheterized, and thus multiple potential sites of occlusion (e.g., anterior vs. posterior circulation) can be accessed.

Procedure Technique

Using a transfemoral approach, with the Seldinger technique, and prior to placement of the Introducer sheath, we place a percutaneous Perclose ProGlide Suture-Mediated Closure (SMC) System (Abbott Vascular), which is left untied and knotted at the end of the procedure after removing the Introducer sheath.

An 8 Fr balloon guide catheter is placed in the proximal ICA for the carotid territory and the subclavian artery for the vertebrobasilar territory. We consider a fundamental part of this technique the use of a balloon guide catheter, because it allows the anterograde flow to stop by making the arterial occlusion and also allows it to reverse the flow through aspiration, increasing efficiency in the extraction of the thrombus and preventing the migration of fragments of the thrombus to other vascular territories.

A heparin bolus is not administered, and no heparinized saline solution is continuously perfused through the catheter during the procedure.

With the balloon of the guide catheter deflated, a 0.014 inch guidewire is advanced through the clot (with the tip bent) within the occluded intracranial vessel. The 18 microcatheter is then advanced over this wire through the clot, and the guidewire is exchanged for the embolectomy device (retrievable stent). Then, the retrievable stent is advanced and deployed over the clot with the distal portion of the stent placed a few millimeters away from the clot, opening the vessel and allowing blood flow in the lenticulostriate and distal branches if the clot length is shorter than the stent (in almost all cases we used a retrievable stent that was 4 × 20 mm, but with the advent of longer retrievable stents we have started using 4 × 40 mm stents). To prevent arterial rupture, the distal part of the device is deployed in a straight portion of the artery.

The retrievable stent is kept deployed for 1 to 3 minutes before retrieving in order to better entrap the clot (however; some companies do not recommend waiting, as with the pressure exerted by the retrievable stent by compressing the thrombus against the wall of the vessel, the stent becomes dehydrated and adheres to the arterial wall). The balloon of the guide catheter is then inflated, and the microcatheter and the embolectomy device are gently withdrawn into the body of the guide catheter while aspiration is performed with a 60 mL syringe or suction pump, such as the Penumbra System. The clot is retrieved, and the balloon is then deflated.

Control angiography is then performed to confirm recanalization and reperfusion (▶ Fig. 7.13).

In case the recanalization of the artery is not achieved, several passes are made following the same technique. No pass limit has been described. We usually do not make more than seven passes

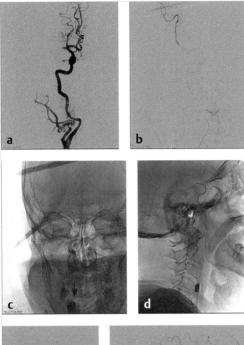

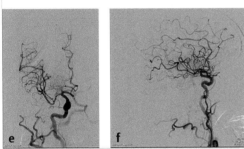

Fig. 7.13 Photographic sequence of the technique of a transfemoral mechanical thrombectomy, of an occlusion of the MCA.

with the same device and instead try other techniques or devices to try to recanalize the vessel.

Tandem Occlusion

If the patient has a tandem occlusion, we do a small angioplasty (with a balloon 2 × 20 mm) to allow passage of the balloon guide catheter before distal MT. Once the ICA is catheterized, the MT is performed with the technique described above. After intracranial recanalization, we peform an angioplasty of the ICA (with a balloon 5 × 20 mm). Prior to ICA angioplasty, we occlude the CCA with the balloon-guide catheter and perform the ICA angioplasty under continuous aspiration (▶ Fig. 7.14).

We try to avoid placing a stent to prevent early antiplatelet therapy and hemorrhagic transformation (in accordance with our previous study[26]).

If there is an unstable plaque or a recoil of the stenosis, stenting after thrombectomy is performed in the ICA at the end of the procedure. We never place the stent prior to MT, because the stent retriever can become entangled with the carotid stent, as has been reported.[27]

7.5.2 Transcervical Access

Age and traditional cerebrovascular risk factors promote the elongation and tortuosity of the femoral, iliac, aortic, brachiocephalic, and cervical arteries. Additional challenges in catheter navigation include thoracic aortic aneurysms and severe thoracic aortic atherosclerosis. Therefore, once groin access is achieved, procedural times may be significantly prolonged in cases of difficult anatomy. Sometimes the target vessel cannot be quickly catheterized, or is impossible to catheterize, via the transfemoral approach, necessitating alternative access via a transcervical approach.

Procedure Technique

In the supine position, the neck is extended. A rolled sheet is placed underneath the shoulders to help facilitate positioning. The neck is sterilized with an iodine povidone solution and then prepped and draped in normal sterile fashion. After subcutaneous administration of 2% lidocaine, the left CCA is visualized with ultrasonography (US) as necessary to achieve access using an Abbocath needle. The most superficial aspect of the CCA proximal to the bifurcation is targeted. Once brisk arterial blood is visualized in the Abbocath needle, an angled 0.035 guidewire is advanced, followed by a 6 Fr Introducer sheath with the Seldinger technique.

A skin incision is necessary to facilitate catheter advancement. It should be noted that advancing the sheath through the cervical carotid is much more difficult than penetrating the femoral artery and requires significant forward pressure. The Introducer sheath is subsequently connected to a pressurized non-heparinized saline infusion. The introducer sheath was advanced as distally as possible over the wire.

From this point of the procedure, the technique with a retrievable stent can be used as described above, or the ADAPT technique can be used (as we have also previously described[25] and as described elsewhere in this book).

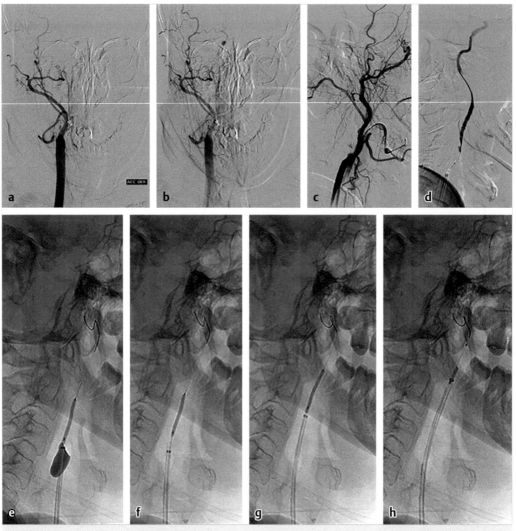

Fig. 7.14 **(a-h)** Photographic sequence of the technique of a transfemoral mechanical thrombectomy, of a tandem occlusion.

Finally, we closed the carotid access point with a percutaneous closure.

While transcervical access may facilitate faster and higher rates of recanalization in a subset of patients, many challenges remain. The most important is difficulty achieving hemostasis, with resultant neck hematoma. This can lead to elective intubation for airway protection, although surgical hematoma evacuation is not always necessary. Previous series have reported a 4 to 7% rate of neck hematoma after introducer sheath removal.[28] An open surgical exposure may be superior in achieving hemostasis, as it mitigates the need for manual compression or a closure device; however, open surgical exposure may not be readily feasible in the acute stroke setting. Although manual compression alone has also been used with good success, even in cases of patients on dual antiplatelet therapy[29] at present, the use of closure devices for this technique is limited but has a promising future. The ideal closure device would be exclusively extravascular and would avoid the need for leaving behind an intravascular foreign body with subsequent risk of distal embolization. However, a previous paper described the use of the Mynx closure device (Access Closure, Inc) without good success for carotid artery closure.[30] The use of alternative transfemoral closure devices such as

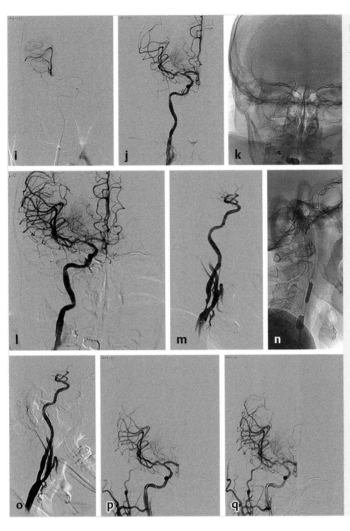

Fig. 9.14 *(continued)* **(i-q)** Photographic sequence of the technique of a transfemoral mechanical thrombectomy, of a tandem occlusion.

Angio-Seal (St. Jude's Medical, Inc)[31] and StarClose (Abbott) may lead to superior results. The use of Perclose ProGlide (Abbott) or Exoseal (Cordis) for this purpose has not been described.

In the author's institution, we use the Angio-Seal Evolution vascular closure device (St. Jude Medical), with excellent results.[25]

7.6 Complications of this Technique

In this section, we will describe the complications of this technique and some guides or tricks to avoid them.

This technique, like any other, is not exempt from complications, but fortunately, the complication rate is very low, as summarized in the table below (▶ Table 7.1).

- **Embolism in another territory that has been treated**

This complication may occur in particular because of two circumstances:

a) The thrombus, which has been caught with the retrievable stent, fractions during the extraction maneuvers, and a portion of the thrombus leaps into another territory (e.g., a fragment of a thrombus in the MCA jumps to ACA during during the mechanical thrombectomy (MT), or

b) A thrombus or plaque fragment of the nutritional artery Internal Carotid Artery (ICA) or Vertebral Artery (VA) jumps to another territory other than the location of the thrombus intended to be treated during maneuvers involved in the MT.

How to avoid it:

Table 7.1 Comparative table of complications in the five randomized studies

	MR CLEAN	EXTEN-IA	ESCAPE	SWIF PRIME	REVASCAT
Embolization in another territory	20/233 (8, 6%)	2/35 (6%)	-	-	5/103 (4, 9%)
Dissection of an arterial vessel	4/233 (1, 7%)	-	-	-	4/103 (3, 9%)
Perforation of an arterial vessel	2/233 (0, 9%)	2/35 (6%)	1/165 (9, 6%)	3/98 (3%)	5/103 (4, 9%)
Hematoma at the puncture site	-	1/35 (3%) (Required transfusion)	3/165 (1, 8%)	-	11/103 (10, 7%)
Pseudoaneurysm at the puncture site	-	-	-	-	1/103 (3, 9%)
Vasospasm requiring treatment	-	-	-	4/98 (4%)	4/103 (3, 9%)
Symptomatic cerebral hematoma	There were no significant differences in any of the trials with the control group				
Unwanted detachment of the Solitaire	None of these trials describes this complication				

- ○ Perform the occlusion with the balloon-guide catheter.
- ○ Provide continuous aspiration.

- **Perforation or arterial dissection**

This is one of the complications that most influence the technique used.

Because the catheterization of the occluded arteries is done blindly, since the thrombus prevents the passage of contrast, it must be performed gently and carefully, avoiding force when there is difficulty passing the guidewire or the microcatheter.

How to avoid it:

- ○ Perform the catheterization with the distal end of the guidewire bent.

  In the author's experience, we have occasionally found an aneurysm after the thrombus has been removed, and almost certainly, if we had not passed the guidewire with its distal end bent, we would have pierced the aneurysm.

- ○ Leave the distal end of the microcatheter in a straight portion of the artery to deploy the retrievable stent.

- **Hematoma at the puncture site**:

Because MT is performed by vascular access of important arteries, such as the femoral or carotid artery, and with large-caliber sheath introducers, in patients who may have received IV thrombolysis there is a very significant risk of hematomas developing at the site of puncture.

How to avoid it:

- ○ Use percutaneous closure.

- **Unwanted detachment of the Solitaire**:

Spontaneous detachment of the stent may also occur owing to fatigue of the material due to prolonged use, additional stress from the technique used, damage during washing for reuse, or a manufacturing defect.

Unwanted spontaneous detachment of the stent during clot retrieval was classified as proximal to the stent proximal marker (type A) or distal to the marker (type B). This procedural complication was reported with a rate of 2.3%, and was associated with a higher number of retrieval attempts and resulted in a significant increase in sICH and poor clinical outcome.[32]

In these cases, we attempted to capture the device with an Amplatz GooseNeck Snare (Medtronic). Once the stent was gripped by the loop, we proceeded to extract it, using the same technique as described earlier to remove the thrombus. Our results show that type A detachment can be recovered, whereas type B is almost impossible to recapture. This might be because in type A detachment, the proximal marker remains attached to the stent and makes the stent's legs converge and join the marker. This allows a radiopaque reference to direct the snare and slide it around the stent to capture the Solitaire. In the B type, the break occurs at the junction of the stent with the proximal marker, allowing the stent's legs to open or stay together, making a spearhead-like shape that digs into the wall of the artery. In this situation, there is no radiopaque reference to direct the snare, and as the stent's legs are leaning against the arterial wall, it becomes very difficult to slide the loop out of the stent to capture the Solitaire.[32]

How to avoid it:

- ○ Protect the proximal part of the stent with the distal end of the microcatheter.
- ○ Use new-generation retrievable stents with reinforcement at the junction with the guidewire.
- ○ It is possible that there is a greater risk of this complication with the Solumbra technique.
- **Hemorrhagic transformation**:
  This is a known complication of ischemic stroke that may occur independently of MT and depends on multiple factors (ischemia time, infarct size, etc.), although there are some factors related to MT which may increase or facilitate it, such as increased blood flow after opening the arteries or administration of drugs that alter coagulation mechanisms (antiplatelet agents, fibrinolytics, heparin), etc.
  How to avoid it:
- ○ Do not use heparin.
- ○ Try not to use (release) a carotid stent or intracranial stent in the acute phase. (Because double antiaggregation is required).
- ○ Make a rigorous selection of patients who will be treated with this technique.

7.7 Conclusion

The development of new techniques and strategies for recanalization has evolved so much in recent years that it has been a revolution in the treatment of stroke. The introduction of new techniques such as retrievable stents and ADAPT have drastically changed the results described above. Currently, recanalization is not only obtained at much higher rates than those obtained with the previous techniques, it is also performed faster. This increase in recanalization has been accompanied by a clinical benefit for patients, 33 to 71% of whom reach functional independence (mRS ≤ 2) (MR CLEAN 32,6%, REVASCAT 43,7%, EASCAPE 53%, SWIFT PRIME 60%, EXTEND-IA 71%) at 3 months, compared to 25–46% described by previous series. However, there is still a lot of work to be done and a lot of problems to solve—accurate and reproducible diagnostic techniques in all regions of a country; fast patient transfer networks from any part of a region to centers with high technology; neuroprotective drugs to be used from the first symptoms until the treatment, etc.,)—and it is necessary to develop new techniques that allow us to recanalize patients who cannot be treated with current devices.

References

[1] Smith WS, Furlan AJ. Brief History of Endovascular Acute Ischemic Stroke Treatment. Stroke. 2016; 47(2):e23–e26

[2] Zeumer H, Hacke W, Ringelstein EB. Local intraarterial thrombolysis in vertebrobasilar thromboembolic disease. AJNR Am J Neuroradiol. 1983; 4(3):401–404

[3] del Zoppo GJ, Higashida RT, Furlan AJ, Pessin MS, Rowley HA, Gent M. PROACT: a phase II randomized trial of recombinant pro-urokinase by direct arterial delivery in acute middle cerebral artery stroke. PROACT Investigators. Prolyse in Acute Cerebral Thromboembolism. Stroke. 1998; 29(1):4–11

[4] Furlan A, Higashida R, Wechsler L, et al. Intra-arterial prourokinase for acute ischemic stroke. The PROACT II study: a randomized controlled trial. Prolyse in Acute Cerebral Thromboembolism. JAMA. 1999; 282(21):2003–2011

[5] http://radiology.ucla.edu/merci-retriever

[6] Smith WS, Sung G, Starkman S, et al. MERCI Trial Investigators. Safety and efficacy of mechanical embolectomy in acute ischemic stroke: results of the MERCI trial. Stroke. 2005; 36 (7):1432–1438

[7] Smith WS, Sung G, Saver J, et al. Multi MERCI Investigators. Mechanical thrombectomy for acute ischemic stroke: final results of the Multi MERCI trial. Stroke. 2008; 39(4):1205–1212

[8] Bose A, Henkes H, Alfke K, et al. Penumbra Phase 1 Stroke Trial Investigators. The Penumbra system: a mechanical device for the treatment of acute stroke due to thromboembolism. AJNR Am J Neuroradiol. 2008; 29:409–413

[9] Desk R, Williams L, Health K, Penumbra Pivotal Stroke Trial Investigators. The penumbra pivotal stroke trial: safety and effectiveness of a new generation of mechanical devices for clot removal in intracranial large vessel occlusive disease. Stroke. 2009; 40(8):2761–2768

[10] Tarr R, Hsu D, Kulcsar Z, et al. The POST trial: initial postmarket experience of the Penumbra system: revascularization of large vessel occlusion in acute ischemic stroke in the United States and Europe. J Neurointerv Surg. 2010; 2(4):341–344

[11] Turk AS, Frei D, Fiorella D, et al. ADAPT FAST study: a direct aspiration first pass technique for acute stroke thrombectomy. J Neurointerv Surg. 2014; 6(4):260–264

[12] Liebig T, Henkes H, Reinartz J, Miloslavski E, Kühne D. A novel self-expanding fully retrievable intracranial stent (SOLO): experience in nine procedures of stent-assisted aneurysm coil occlusion. Neuroradiology. 2006; 48(7):471–478

[13] Castaño C, Serena J, Dávalos A. Use of the New Solitaire (TM) AB Device for Mechanical Thrombectomy when Merci Clot Retriever Has Failed to Remove the Clot. A Case Report. Interv Neuroradiol. 2009; 15(2):209–214

[14] Castaño C, Dorado L, Guerrero C, et al. Mechanical thrombectomy with the Solitaire AB device in large artery occlusions of the anterior circulation: a pilot study. Stroke. 2010; 41(8):1836–1840

[15] Saver JL, Jahan R, Levy EI, et al. SWIFT Trialists. Solitaire flow restoration device versus the Merci Retriever in patients with acute ischaemic stroke (SWIFT): a randomised, parallel-group, non-inferiority trial. Lancet. 2012; 380(9849):1241–1249

[16] Pereira VM, Gralla J, Davalos A, et al. Prospective, multicenter, single-arm study of mechanical thrombectomy using Solitaire Flow Restoration in acute ischemic stroke. Stroke. 2013; 44(10):2802–2807

[17] Berkhemer OA, Fransen PS, Beumer D, et al. MR CLEAN Investigators. A randomized trial of intraarterial treatment for acute ischemic stroke. N Engl J Med. 2015; 372(1):11–20

[18] Campbell BC, Mitchell PJ, Kleinig TJ, et al. EXTEND-IA Investigators. Endovascular therapy for ischemic stroke with perfusion-imaging selection. N Engl J Med. 2015; 372(11): 1009–1018

[19] Goyal M, Demchuk AM, Menon BK, et al. ESCAPE Trial Investigators. Randomized assessment of rapid endovascular treatment of ischemic stroke. N Engl J Med. 2015; 372(11):1019–1030

[20] Saver JL, Goyal M, Bonafe A, et al. SWIFT PRIME Investigators. Stent-retriever thrombectomy after intravenous t-PA vs. t-PA alone in stroke. N Engl J Med. 2015; 372(24):2285–2295

[21] Jovin TG, Chamorro A, Cobo E, et al. REVASCAT Trial Investigators. Thrombectomy within 8 hours after symptom onset in ischemic stroke. N Engl J Med. 2015; 372(24):2296–2306

[22] Soares BP, Chien JD, Wintermark M. MR and CT monitoring of recanalization, reperfusion, and penumbra salvage: everything that recanalizes does not necessarily reperfuse! Stroke. 2009; 40(3) Suppl:S24–S27

[23] Protocolos de Neurointervencionismo y de Tratamiento Trombolítico en Situaciones Especiales en el Ictus Isquémico Agudo. Servicios de Neurología, Radiodiagnóstico, IDI (Institut Diagnòstic per Imatge) y Neurorradiología intervencionista de los hospitales: Hospital Universitario Germans Trias i Pujol, Badalona, Hospital Doctor Josep Trueta, Girona, Hospital del Mar, Barcelona. Enero 2009. ISBN 978-84-691-9848-3

[24] European Stroke Organisation (ESO) Executive Committee, ESO Writing Committee. Guidelines for management of ischaemic stroke and transient ischaemic attack 2008. Cerebrovasc Dis. 2008; 25(5):457–507

[25] Castaño C, Remollo S, García MR, Hidalgo C, Hernández-Perez M, Ciorba M. Mechanical thrombectomy with 'ADAPT' technique by transcervical access in acute ischemic stroke. Neuroradiol J. 2015; 28(6):617–622

[26] Dorado L, Castaño C, Millán M, et al. Hemorrhagic risk of emergent endovascular treatment plus stenting in patients with acute ischemic stroke. J Stroke Cerebrovasc Dis. 2013; 22(8):1326–1331

[27] Miteff F, Faulder KC, Goh AC, Steinfort BS, Sue C, Harrington TJ. Mechanical thrombectomy with a self-expanding retrievable intracranial stent (Solitaire AB): experience in 26 patients with acute cerebral artery occlusion. AJNR Am J Neuroradiol. 2011; 32(6):1078–1081

[28] Blanc R, Piotin M, Mounayer C, Spelle L, Moret J. Direct cervical arterial access for intracranial endovascular treatment. Neuroradiology. 2006; 48(12):925–929

[29] Mathieu X, Piret V, Bergeron P, Petrosyan A, Abdulamit T, Trastour JC. Choice of access for percutaneous carotid angioplasty and stenting: a comparative study on cervical and femoral access. J Cardiovasc Surg (Torino). 2009; 50(5):677–681

[30] Jadhav AP, Ribo M, Grandhi R, et al. Transcervical access in acute ischemic stroke. J Neurointerv Surg. 2014; 6(9):652–657

[31] Blanc R, Mounayer C, Piotin M, Sadik JC, Spelle L, Moret J. Hemostatic closure device after carotid puncture for stent and coil placement in an intracranial aneurysm: technical note. AJNR Am J Neuroradiol. 2002; 23(6):978–981

[32] Castaño C, Dorado L, Remollo S, et al. Unwanted detachment of the Solitaire device during mechanical thrombectomy in acute ischemic stroke. J Neurointerv Surg. 2016; 8(12):1226–1230

8 Direct Aspiration Thrombectomy for Acute Stroke: Evolution of Technique and Evidence

Alejandro M. Spiotta and Aquilla S. Turk

Abstract

Thrombectomy techniques for achieving recanalization of an occluded large vessel occlusion have undergone rapid advances since the first approved device. The first techniques were modestly effective and entailed long procedure times. Newer approaches over the last several years have resulted in very high rates of successful recanalization and increasingly faster procedure times. This chapter reviews the mechanics and rationale for the evolution of thrombectomy approaches and provides a summary of the latest evidence in support of the latest generation thrombectomy technique, direct aspiration.

Keywords: thrombectomy, technique, evolution, stent retriever, direct aspiration

8.1 Introduction

Under mounting pressure to have evidence in support of thrombectomy over iv-tPA, five randomized controlled trials[1,2,3,4,5] were launched shortly after the release of the negative trials of 2013. An impressive collective effort and rapid enrollment culminated in the halting of the trials in 2015 due to overwhelming statistical efficacy of thrombectomy over medical management. That year marked the largest improvement in therapeutic options for acute ischemic stroke care since the NINDs trial in 1995 and armed us for the first time with a mechanical thrombectomy device, the stent retriever (SR), with level 1A evidence supporting its use. We now detail the origins and technical nuances of the next-generation thrombectomy approach: direct aspiration.

8.2 Direct Aspiration

Acute stroke thrombectomy approaches have evolved rapidly. Spurred primarily by advances in catheter technology as well as the thrombectomy device itself, we are now able to achieve higher recanalization rates than ever before. We review the key technological advances and design modifications that have allowed for navigation around the ophthalmic turn for more distal delivery of larger-bore catheters providing more aspiration force directly applied at the thrombus interface.

8.2.1 Direct Aspiration Origins: the Penumbra 054 Aspiration Catheter

The Penumbra aspiration system introduced in 2008 involved maceration of the thrombus with a separator which was repeatedly introduced and withdrawn from the thrombus under direct aspiration to prevent showering of fragments.[6] While its market competitor at the time, the Merci system, relied primarily on delivery of a microcatheter (the 18 L; Stryker) to the site of occlusion, the Penumbra aspiration system relied on the delivery of a much larger bore catheter to the thrombus (up to effectively a 5 F device). The introduction of highly flexible lubricious polymers with good hoop strength allowed for safe placement of large intermediate class catheters directly into the large intracranial vessels. The development of large-bore flexible catheters was essential to the function of the Penumbra system.

The original iteration of the Penumbra reperfusion catheter system included several different sized catheters (internal diameter 0.026", 0.032", and 0.041") and accompanying separators to maximize clot interaction and force of aspiration in vessels of differing diameters (internal carotid artery terminus, M1, M2, M3) to address both proximal and distal thrombi.[7] The largest catheter at the time of first launch had a lumen diameter of 0.041 inch, yet it tracked suboptimally around the carotid siphon and required a median 45 minutes to achieve acceptable recanalization min.[8] In 2009, the Reperfusion Catheter 054 became available, which dramatically improved the aspiration efficiency to a median 20 minutes[8] due to its much larger tapered lumen. As the aspiration force is proportional to the square of the diameter of the catheter, the 054 catheter provided an estimated 4× aspiration force over the next smaller catheter, the 041.[8]

Although a larger catheter lumen provides higher suction and more rapid removal of thrombus, a drawback of its larger size was that the 054 catheter often required the use of a coaxial technique to facilitate navigation to the middle cerebral artery. When navigated over a 0.014 inch microwire alone, a significant ledge would get held up at the origin of the ophthalmic artery. To overcome this obstacle to the target lesion, access with the 054 catheter could be optimized with a coaxial technique (▶ Fig. 8.1). The smaller 032 and 026 reperfusion catheters could be delivered simply over either a 0.014 or 0.016 inch wire, and the larger 054 delivered over those. One of the major advantages of the Penumbra aspiration system was that once the catheter system was delivered to the target vessel, separator clot maceration could be performed without having to re-access (additional 'passes'), as was the case for the Merci device.[9]

Despite these advances in catheter technology, navigating past the carotid siphon was still a relative challenge during thrombectomy cases. In patients with very acute angulation in the ophthalmic segment, adjunctive techniques could be performed to obtain the necessary distal access. One approach used the Merci Retriever System (Concentric Medical) as an adjunct to improve the trackability of the 054 reperfusion catheter by altering the angle with which the catheter engages the ophthalmic segment and M1 origin. By deploying an appropriately-sized Merci Retriever, such as a V.2.0 or V.2.5 soft, in the mid M1 segment through either the 032 catheter or an 18 L microcatheter and then applying gentle traction on the Merci Retriever, the course of the wire straightens, approximating the inner curve of the vasculature, pulling the catheter complex away from the ledge of the vessel origins ("grappling hook" technique),[10,11] an approach now used routinely using SRs and intermediate catheters. The 054 catheter can then be more readily advanced into the target vessel. Once the 054 reperfusion catheter is in place, the retriever is resheathed into the 18 L microcatheter and then removed prior to separator placement and aspiration.

The next iteration of the Penumbra aspiration catheter family (Max series) was introduced in 2012 and also intended to be used with separators of varying size. The Max series catheters included larger inner diameters at the distal end as well as the proximal end to increase the aspiration power. The larger proximal lumen reduces resistance to low and therefore increases aspiration force at the catheter tip. Improvements in polymer and braid

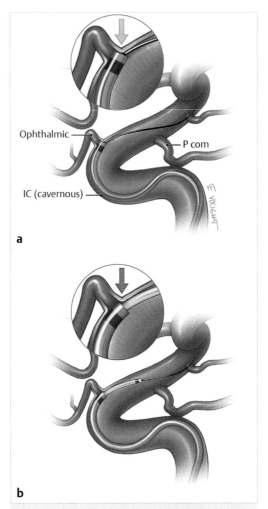

Ophthalmic

P com

IC (cavernous)

a

b

Fig. 8.1 (a) While a larger catheter lumen provides higher suction and more rapid removal of thrombus, it results in a larger catheter profile and "ledge effect" which renders navigation past the ophthalmic artery origin challenging. (b) To overcome this obstacle, access with an intermediate catheter is optimized with a coaxial technique, resulting in a more tapered construct that minimizes the ledge effect.

and ring reinforcement provide more catheter tip flexibility and an increased number of transition zones to improve trackability while maintaining hoop strength. The newly introduced intermediate catheters were named 5Max, 4Max, and 3Max. An increased number of transition zones in the catheter design and manufacturing allowed these catheters to be delivered primarily over either a 0.014 or 0.016 inch microwire, even past the ophthalmic origin.

8.2.2 Direct Aspiration Origins: the Distal Access Catheter

In 2004, the Merci Retriever became the first mechanical thrombectomy device cleared for human use in the United States by the FDA.[12] The Merci device primarily works by engaging the thrombus with a "corkscrew" distal wire and suture tip deployed from within the clot, then removing the thrombus en bloc to achieve recanalization. The device was employed using a balloon-guide catheter that was positioned at the carotid bifurcation or internal carotid artery to cause temporary flow reversal, allowing the Merci to be retrieved into the guide catheter while mitigating the possibility of emboli showering to distal territories. However, clot retrieval into the guide catheter still required a long distance to be traveled while maintaining purchase on the thrombus, most commonly from the M1 segment of the middle cerebral artery to the proximal cervical internal carotid artery. The vector force applied while pulling on the thrombus was suboptimal (downwards along the long axis of the cervical carotid artery, not horizontally along the axis of the middle cerebral artery). This caused considerable torqueing, stretching, and distortion of the parent vessel and presented a biomechanical disadvantage to thrombus removal, as well as traction on the vasculature, resulting in pain for the patient. To avoid the inevitable movement induced, many operators chose to perform thrombectomy under general anesthesia. In addition, the Merci technique required a long distance to be traveled while remaining engaged with the thrombus.

A landmark advancement came in 2010 with the approval of the Outreach Distal Access Catheter (DAC; Concentric Medical), which would have repercussions for the application of the Merci device and also for future iterations of thrombectomy approaches. The DAC was designed for the purpose of buttressing access for the Merci thrombectomy device, affording stable access to the target vessel. Use of the DAC optimized the vectors at play during pulling of the device. With further understanding of clot fragmentation and distal embolization, the DAC was used as an intermediate aspiration device which aided in preventing showering of distal emboli during clot retrieval, increased the aspiration power applied directly to the thrombus.[10,13] The development of large-bore flexible catheters that could be delivered into the intracranial circulation represented a major advance in thrombectomy technology and also in intermediate catheter technology.[13,14] The DAC has a flexible distal shaft with increased proximal shaft strength and axial load-bearing characteristics as well as good hoop strength, allowing it to be delivered to the intracranial circulation around the ophthalmic bend when navigated over a coaxial catheter system. A major drawback to the Merci Retrieval System was that it necessitated navigating past the ophthalmic bend with every pass, decreasing the efficiency of the system and adding to procedure times.

8.3 Current Generation Aspiration: "Solumbra" Technique

Another key milestone in the evolution of thrombectomy technique was developed in the early stages of widespread SR incorporation, the combined SR–penumbra ("Solumbra") technique, which laid the foundation for direct aspiration alone (without the need for a SR). To minimize the distance the SR must travel while engaging the thrombus, especially into larger caliber vasculature such as the internal carotid artery from the middle cerebral artery, and mitigating the possibility of losing purchase of the clot, variations to the SR technique have been employed with incorporation of Penumbra reperfusion catheters. For example, a 5Max catheter can be advanced over a 025 microcatheter and microwire up to the site of occlusion and left at the face of the thrombus. The SR is then deployed, and the microcatheter is removed, leaving the SR in place. The SR is then pulled directly into the 5Max while maintaining aspiration (the so-called "Solumbra" technique, since it combines a stent retriever (Solitaire) with a Penumbra aspiration catheter), and both are removed together (► Fig. 8.2), much in the same way as the Merci retriever device was removed with a DAC. However, traction is minimized as compared with the Merci system, since the force vectors are horizontal in orientation from the aperture of the aspiration catheter in parallel to the M1. This eliminated the painful stimulus that patients were formerly experiencing. Thus, in addition to representing a more effective technique, the now-painless procedure had the added advantage of reintroducing the concept of the awake thrombectomy, with many operators now electing to perform the procedure with minimal conscious sedation. Advantages included the ability to examine the patient's neurological status throughout the procedure,

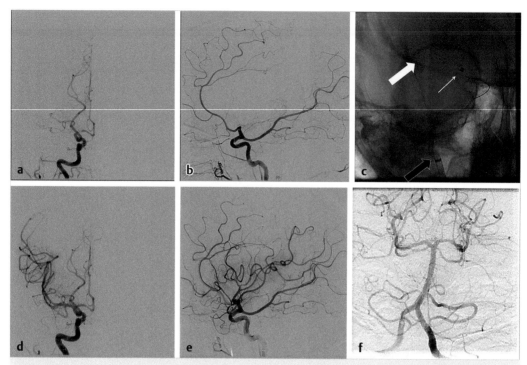

Fig. 8.2 "Solumbra" (Solitaire and Penumbra) technique. **(a)** Anteroposterior (AP) and **(b)** lateral digital subtraction angiography (DSA) demonstrates an M1 occlusion. **(c)** A Solitaire stent retriever (SR) is deployed across the M1 segment occlusion (large white arrow), with the aspiration catheter in the proximal M1 segment (small white arrow) and the guide catheter in the distal cervical internal carotid artery (black arrow). **(d)** The SR is then withdrawn back into the aspiration catheter under direct aspiration applied locally at the M1. The operator may choose to withdraw the SR entirely into the aspiration catheter, or to partially withdraw and then pull both the SR and the aspiration catheter together back to the guide catheter. Aspiration can also be applied at the guide catheter. Some may choose to perform this technique with a balloon guide catheter to affect flow reversal for added protection against distal emboli in the event of thrombus fragmentation. **(e)** AP and lateral DSA demonstrate recanalization of the M1 occlusion (TICI 2B) with showering of distal fragments and small vessel occlusions.

shorter CT-to-groin-stick times, and avoiding the imminent risk of systemic hypotension from induction of general anesthesia.

SR technology was employed exclusively in the ESCAPE, EXTEND-IA, SWIFT PRIME and REVASCAT trials. While the MR CLEAN trial did not dictate which thrombectomy device was to be utilized, the majority of cases were also SR-based. Given that SRs were used in the overwhelming majority of patients enrolled in the positive trials, they have often been referred to as the "stent retriever trials", which is reflected in the updated American Heart Association/American Stroke Association guidelines recommending thrombectomy to be performed with an SR. However, thrombectomy techniques evolved even while those trials were enrolling, setting the stage for the next generation strategy as detailed below.

8.4 Next Generation: Direct Aspiration

Direct aspiration[15,16,17,18] has become possible due to advances in catheter technology that allow large-caliber aspiration catheters to be advanced intracranially to the thrombus. In general, the largest size aspiration catheter that the vessel can accommodate should be utilized. In the first iteration, this was most commonly a Penumbra 5Max Reperfusion Catheter (Penumbra) for M1 or carotid terminus occlusions. The 5Max can be advanced to the level of the thrombus over any microcatheter and microwire the operator choses, but most commonly a Velocity microcatheter (Penumbra) over a 0.016 inch Fathom wire (Boston Scientific Corp). The microcatheter and wire are removed, and aspiration is applied by either a 20 or 60 mL syringe or use of the Penumbra aspiration pump that is part of the Penumbra thrombectomy/aspiration system.[19] Inability to draw back blood on aspiration confirms optimal position of the 5Max catheter abutting the thrombus. The next iteration involved advancing the catheter slightly to ensure firm engagement with the thrombus. The 5Max catheter is then slowly withdrawn while maintaining aspiration. Aspiration is also applied to the sideport of the guide catheter to prevent dislodging the thrombus from the 5Max aperture as it is withdrawn into the sheath. Clots are typically removed en bloc, minimizing the risk of downstream emboli (▶ Fig. 8.3). When this technique is successful, it eliminates the need to introduce SR or penumbra separator devices, leading to an overall much lower procedure device cost.[15,16] Thus, we have found the initial application of this technique to provide the highest cost-effective value in acute stroke treatment.

This approach was facilitated by the development of the Penumbra Max aspiration catheter technology, which significantly increased the ease and speed of navigation of a large-bore catheter into the intracranial circulation. The direct aspiration technique differs from prior thrombectomy methods, as it focuses on engaging and removing the clot in its entirety rather than the use of the separator that was designed to macerate the thrombus and clear the tip of the aspiration catheter.[20] Historically, due to the challenges with tracking an aspiration catheter into the intracranial circulation, catheters had to be telescoped with other catheters together, or other tricks were employed to advance through the siphon.[9,11,21,22,23] However, the superior trackability of the Penumbra Max catheters has given operators the confidence to attempt direct aspiration alone without the fear that it will be a significant time impediment and danger to the patient if intracranial access is lost. The second iteration of the aspiration catheter, the 5Max ACE, has an increased inner diameter of 0060 at the distal 30 cm, while housing a 0.068 proximal end for larger aspiration forces. Advances in catheter technology would soon follow, allowing for even larger-bore catheters to be safely delivered to the intracranial circulation. With the introduction of the ACE 064 and the ACE 068 (Penumbra), the direct aspiration technique was refined further. Owing to the larger aperture of these catheters, the aspiration catheter

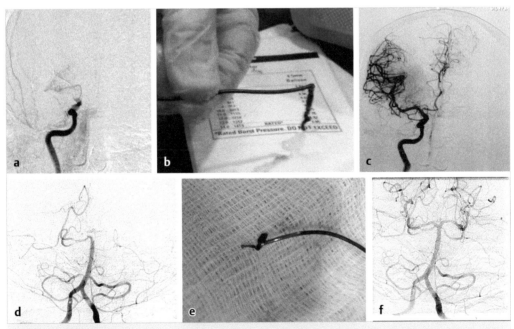

Fig. 8.3 ADAPT illustrations. Direct aspiration typically removed the thrombus en bloc, minimizing the risk of distal emboli. The largest bore aspiration catheter that the occluded vessel will accommodate is advanced to the level of the thrombus. Aspiration is applied to engage the thrombus, which is then removed as demonstrated in the illustrations. **(a-c)** Carotid terminus occlusion recanalized in 15 minutes from groin puncture with direct aspiration thrombectomy in a single pass. **(d-f)** Basilar apex occlusion recanalized in 10 minutes with two passes of direct aspiration thrombectomy.

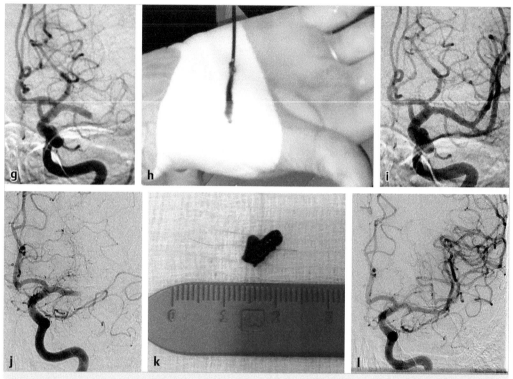

(g-i) MCA bifurcation occlusion recanalized in 12 minutes with a single pass direct aspiration. (j-l) MCA bifurcation occlusion recanalized in 7 minutes with a single pass direct aspiration.

can now be advanced over the thrombus, to "ingest" the thrombus, which is now typically aspirated directly into the catheter without having to remove it (▶ Fig. 8.4).

Another advantage of this approach is that if aspiration alone is not successful at achieving revascularization of the occluded vessel, the Penumbra aspiration catheter can also function as a distal conduit for other devices, such as a smaller 3Max catheter for direct aspiration in more distal branches (M2, P2 or P3, for example), SRs, balloons, or stents. This forms the basis of A Direct Aspiration First Pass Technique (ADAPT) which is gaining in popularity. If direct aspiration attempts are unsuccessful, other attempts, including SR thrombectomy, can then be performed. At the time of writing, two randomized controlled trials of anterior circulation LVO treated within six hours of symptom onset (ASTER, COMPASS) have recently reported noninferiority of ADAPT compared to an SR as the primary modality.[24] While 90-day outcomes were equivalent, ADAPT was associated with faster recanalization times and lower procedural costs.[25]

The newest iteration of direct aspiration involves its application in more distal vasculature. In smaller caliber vessels, the technique can be employed with either a 4Max or 3Max reperfusion catheter (Penumbra). In principle, the largest bore catheter that the occluded vessel can accommodate is selected for aspiration (▶ Fig. 8.5), with effective (TICI ≥ 2B 97.1%) and fast recanalization (mean 35.7 minutes) achieved safely.[17]

8.5 Conclusion

There have been rapid advances in thrombectomy devices and approaches over the past decade, from rudimentary mechanical disruption, followed by intra-arterial thrombolytic infusions to increasingly effective thrombectomy devices (▶ Fig. 8.6).[26] Ongoing improvements in the devices and techniques are yielding improved angiographic and clinical outcomes, allowing patients to enjoy the best outcomes following LVO in recorded history. Device technology, selection strategies, and medical management will likely evolve in tandem, and we look forward to the continued evolution of

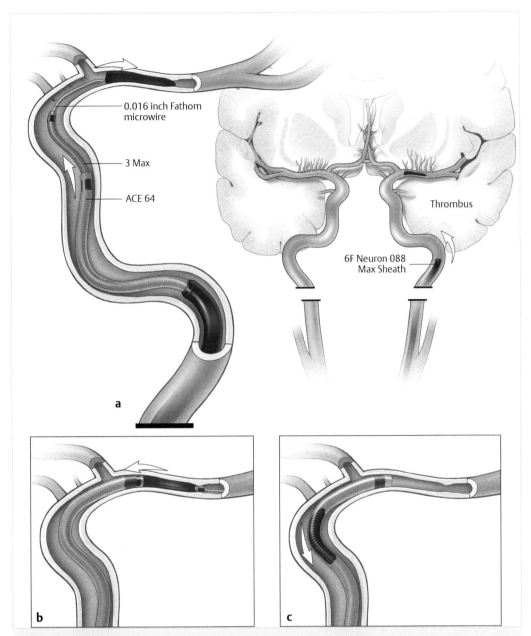

Fig. 8.4 Aspiration catheter technology has rapidly advanced. With the introduction of the ACE 064 and the ACE 068 (Penumbra, Oakland CA), the direct aspiration technique has been refined further. Owing to the larger aperture of these catheters, the aspiration catheter can now be advanced directly over the thrombus to "ingest" the thrombus under aspiration. The thrombus is now typically aspirated directly into the catheter aspiration tubing without having to remove it.

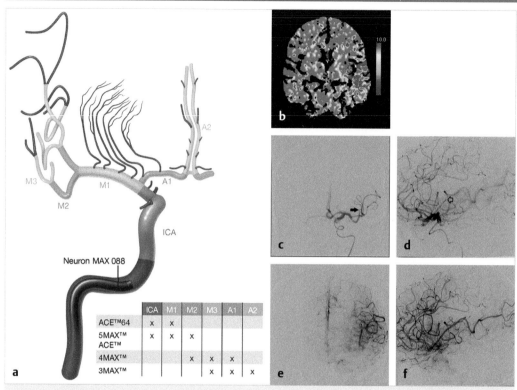

	ICA	M1	M2	M3	A1	A2
ACE™64	x	x				
5MAX™ ACE™	x	x	x			
4MAX™			x	x	x	
3MAX™				x	x	x

Fig. 8.5 (a). Illustration demonstrating aspiration catheter size recommendations for anterior circulation thrombectomy. The guide catheter is positioned in the ICA, providing a platform for thrombectomy with aspiration catheters. (b) CT perfusion imaging demonstrating elevated mean transit time in the left frontal lobe consistent with a left M2 occlusion. (c) AP and (d) lateral projection cerebral angiogram during a left internal carotid injection, demonstrating M2 occlusion with no flow past the site of thrombus (arrows). (e) AP and (f) lateral projection cerebral angiogram during a left internal carotid injection following thrombectomy, demonstrating resolution of M2 occlusion and opacification of distal branches.

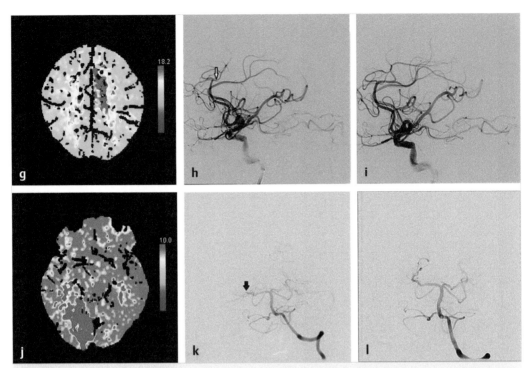

(g) CT perfusion imaging demonstrating elevated mean transit time consistent with a left A2 occlusion. (h) Lateral projection cerebral angiogram demonstrating A2 occlusion (arrow) (i) Postthrombectomy lateral projection cerebral angiogram with resolution of A2 occlusion and complete opacification of distal branches. (j) CT perfusion imaging demonstrating elevated mean transit time in the right occipital lobe consistent with right P2 ischemia. (k) Cerebral angiogram with AP projection from a left vertebral artery injection demonstrating right P2 occlusion and no opacification distal to the thrombus (arrow). (l) Post thrombectomy cerebral angiogram with AP projection from a left vertebral artery injection demonstrating resolution of the thrombus with opacification of the distal PCA branches.

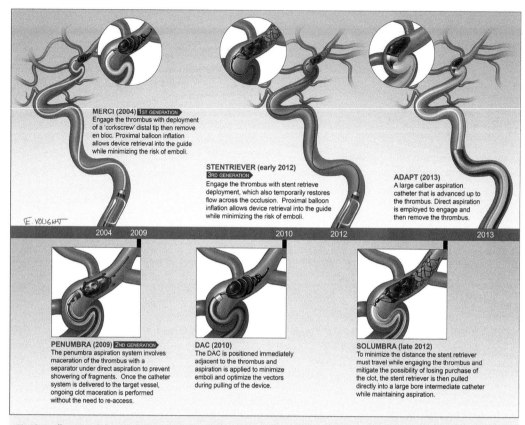

MERCI (2004) 1ST GENERATION
Engage the thrombus with deployment of a 'corkscrew' distal tip then remove en bloc. Proximal balloon inflation allows device retrieval into the guide while minimizing the risk of emboli.

STENTRIEVER (early 2012)
3RD GENERATION
Engage the thrombus with stent retrieve deployment, which also temporarily restores flow across the occlusion. Proximal balloon inflation allows device retrieval into the guide while minimizing the risk of emboli.

ADAPT (2013)
A large caliber aspiration catheter that is advanced up to the thrombus. Direct aspiration is employed to engage and then remove the thrombus.

E. VOUGHT

2004   2009   2010   2012   2013

PENUMBRA (2009) 2ND GENERATION
The penumbra aspiration system involves maceration of the thrombus with a separator under direct aspiration to prevent showering of fragments. Once the catheter system is delivered to the target vessel, ongoing clot maceration is performed without the need to re-access.

DAC (2010)
The DAC is positioned immediately adjacent to the thrombus and aspiration is applied to minimize emboli and optimize the vectors during pulling of the device.

SOLUMBRA (late 2012)
To minimize the distance the stent retriever must travel while engaging the thrombus and mitigate the possibility of losing purchase of the clot, the stent retriever is then pulled directly into a large bore intermediate catheter while maintaining aspiration.

Fig. 8.6 Illustration depicting the major steps in evolution of thrombectomy devices, beginning from the first-generation concept to state-of-the-art approaches.

thrombectomy approaches for acute stroke in the future.

References

[1] Berkhemer OA, Fransen PS, Beumer D, et al. MR CLEAN Investigators. A randomized trial of intraarterial treatment for acute ischemic stroke. N Engl J Med. 2015; 372(1):11–20

[2] Goyal M, Demchuk AM, Menon BK, et al. ESCAPE Trial Investigators. Randomized assessment of rapid endovascular treatment of ischemic stroke. N Engl J Med. 2015; 372(11):1019–1030

[3] Campbell BC, Mitchell PJ, Kleinig TJ, et al. EXTEND-IA Investigators. Endovascular therapy for ischemic stroke with perfusion-imaging selection. N Engl J Med. 2015; 372(11):1009–1018

[4] Saver JL, Goyal M, Bonafe A, et al. SWIFT PRIME Investigators. Stent-retriever thrombectomy after intravenous t-PA vs. t-PA alone in stroke. N Engl J Med. 2015; 372(24):2285–2295

[5] Jovin TG, Chamorro A, Cobo E, et al. REVASCAT Trial Investigators. Thrombectomy within 8 hours after symptom onset in ischemic stroke. N Engl J Med. 2015; 372(24):2296–2306

[6] Nogueira RG, Lutsep HL, Gupta R, et al. TREVO 2 Trialists. Trevo versus Merci retrievers for thrombectomy revascularisation of large vessel occlusions in acute ischaemic stroke (TREVO 2): a randomised trial. Lancet. 2012; 380(9849):1231–1240

[7] Turk AS, Spiotta A, Frei D, et al. Initial clinical experience with the ADAPT technique: A direct aspiration first pass technique for stroke thrombectomy. J Neurointerv Surg. 2013

[8] Turk AS, Campbell JM, Spiotta A, et al. An investigation of the cost and benefit of mechanical thrombectomy for endovascular treatment of acute ischemic stroke. J Neurointerv Surg. 2013

[9] Park MS, Stiefel MF, Fiorella D, Kelly M, McDougall CG, Albuquerque FC. Intracranial placement of a new, compliant guide catheter: technical note. Neurosurgery. 2008; 63(3):E616–E617, discussion E617

[10] Kelly ME, Furlan AJ, Fiorella D. Recanalization of an acute middle cerebral artery occlusion using a self-expanding, reconstrainable, intracranial microstent as a temporary endovascular bypass. Stroke. 2008; 39(6):1770–1773

[11] Chaudhary N, Pandey AS, Thompson BG, Gandhi D, Ansari SA, Gemmete JJ. Utilization of the Neuron 6 French 0.053 inch inner luminal diameter guide catheter for treatment of cerebral vascular pathology: continued experience with ultra distal access into the cerebral vasculature. J Neurointerv Surg. 2012; 4(4):301–306

[12] Frei D, Gerber J, Turk A, et al. The SPEED study: initial clinical evaluation of the Penumbra novel 054 Reperfusion Catheter. J Neurointerv Surg. 2013; 5 Suppl 1:i74–i76

[13] Levy EI, Ecker RD, Horowitz MB, et al. Stent-assisted intracranial recanalization for acute stroke: early results. Neurosurgery. 2006; 58(3):458–463, discussion 458–463

[14] Mocco J, Hanel RA, Sharma J, et al. Use of a vascular reconstruction device to salvage acute ischemic occlusions refractory to traditional endovascular recanalization methods. J Neurosurg. 2010; 112(3):557–562

[15] Turk AS, Frei D, Fiorella D, et al. ADAPT FAST study: a direct aspiration first pass technique for acute stroke thrombectomy. J Neurointerv Surg. 2014; 6(4):260–264

[16] Turk AS, Turner R, Spiotta A, et al. Comparison of endovascular treatment approaches for acute ischemic stroke: cost effectiveness, technical success, and clinical outcomes. J Neurointerv Surg. 2015; 7(9):666–670

[17] Vargas J, Spiotta A, Fargen K, Turner R, Chaudry I, Turk A. Long term experience using the ADAPT technique for the treatment of acute ischemic stroke. J Neurointerv Surg. 2016

[18] Vargas J, Spiotta AM, Fargen K, Turner RD, Chaudry I, Turk A. Experience with ADAPT for Thrombectomy in Distal Cerebral Artery Occlusions Causing Acute Ischemic Stroke. World Neurosurg. 2016

[19] Yoo AJ, Frei D, Tateshima S, et al. The Penumbra Stroke System: a technical review. J Neurointerv Surg. 2012; 4(3):199–205

[20] Tarr R, Hsu D, Kulcsar Z, et al. The POST trial: initial postmarket experience of the Penumbra system: revascularization of large vessel occlusion in acute ischemic stroke in the United States and Europe. J Neurointerv Surg. 2010; 2(4):341–344

[21] Spiotta AM, Hussain MS, Sivapatham T, et al. The versatile distal access catheter: the Cleveland Clinic experience. Neurosurgery. 2011; 68(6):1677–1686, discussion 1686

[22] Turk A, Manzoor MU, Nyberg EM, Turner RD, Chaudry I. Initial experience with distal guide catheter placement in the treatment of cerebrovascular disease: clinical safety and efficacy. J Neurointerv Surg. 2012

[23] Hui FK, Hussain MS, Spiotta A, et al. Merci retrievers as access adjuncts for reperfusion catheters: the grappling hook technique. Neurosurgery. 2012; 70(2):456–460, discussion 460

[24] Lapergue B, Blanc R, Gory B, et al. ASTER Trial Investigators. Effect of Endovascular Contact Aspiration vs Stent Retriever on Revascularization in Patients With Acute Ischemic Stroke and Large Vessel Occlusion: The ASTER Randomized Clinical Trial. JAMA. 2017; 318(5):443–452

[25] Mocco J, Turk ASR, Siddiqui A. A Comparison of direct aspiration vs. stent retriever as a first approach (COMPASS). International Stroke Conference, 2018

[26] Spiotta AM, Chaudry MI, Hui FK, Turner RD, Kellogg RT, Turk AS. Evolution of thrombectomy approaches and devices for acute stroke: a technical review. J Neurointerv Surg. 2015; 7(1):2–7

9 Neuroanesthesia Considerations in Acute Ischemic Stroke

Joseph Whiteley

Abstract

Successfully providing anesthesia for acute ischemic stroke has many challenges. Time sensitive evaluation and management of these critically ill patients is paramount in minimizing ischemic insult. The anesthesiologist must have a thorough understanding of stroke pathology and the interactions of anesthetic agents on cerebral physiology to provide optimal outcomes.

Keywords: ischemia, stroke, cerebral perfusion, cerebral autoregulation, neurophysiology

The anesthesia objectives for revascularization of acute ischemic stroke (AIS) are similar to the goals for many endovascular procedures. Anesthesia provides patient immobility, hemodynamic manipulation, airway protection, intraprocedure neurologic evaluation, medical management, and safe transport of critically ill patients.[1] What makes AIS treatment unique is that it is a neurologic emergency. The primary goal is to restore cerebral blood flow as quickly as possible. Anesthesia services should be adaptable to help achieve this end. The anesthesiologist must often act quickly with limited information. To most effectively care for these patients, the anesthesia provider should be familiar with the pathophysiology of ischemic stroke, manage coexisting disease, understand the effects of anesthetic technique on cerebral physiology, and be able to provide an anesthetic which allows the proceduralist to achieve a successful outcome while minimizing neurologic insult to the patient.

9.1 The Acute Stroke Patient

Providing anesthesia in the neuroendovascular suite can be challenging for a number of reasons. This location is designed to facilitate a wide range of neuroendovascular procedures. However, unlike an operating room, anesthesia is often not involved, and therefore physical space and ergonomic design for anesthesia personnel and equipment is suboptimal.[2] Furthermore, anesthetizing in remote locations can be hazardous. Compared with operating room patients, those receiving anesthesia in remote locations are generally older and sicker. An analysis the American Society of Anesthesiologists (ASA) Closed Claims Project Database reveals adverse respiratory events during monitored anesthesia care in remote nonoperating room locations poses a significant risk to patients.[3] Vigilance and care must be taken to avoid oversedation in this patient population. It is important to maintain the same monitoring standards in the neuroendovascular suite as the operating room.

AIS is a neurologic emergency, and the anesthesia preprocedure evaluation is time limited. Additionally, these patients often present with altered mental status, which makes obtaining a history difficult. However, there are diagnostic tests and patient information that should be acquired before the patient arrives to the endovascular suite. Age, vital signs, allergies, medications, comorbidities, onset of stroke symptoms, and neurologic status, including National Institute of Health Stroke Scale (NIHSS) score, should be known.[4] Recommended test results include EKG, chest X-ray, computed tomography (CT) of vessel occlusion, serum glucose, CBC, platelet count, and coagulation studies.[5] This information, along with a rapid airway evaluation, is often the extent of an anesthesiologist's preprocedure evaluation.

9.2 Airway Management

The decision as to whether a patient will receive conscious sedation or a general anesthetic is often predicated upon the patient's airway patency and their ability to maintain effective ventilation while being positioned supine. If the patient is unable to lie without obstructing their airway, it is prudent to induce general anesthesia and secure the airway before starting the procedure. The anesthesiologist should be able to anticipate potential problems based upon patient characteristics. Male sex, obesity, and sleep apnea are risk factors for difficult mask ventilation.[6,7] Risk factors for difficult tracheal intubation include limited mouth opening, large neck circumference, short thyromental distance, neck immobility, and the inability to visualize the hypopharynx.[8] As neuroendovascular suites are often in a remote location, there should be dedicated difficult intubation equipment readily available.

9.3 Physiologic Monitoring

Monitoring of the AIS patient should meet, at the minimum, ASA standards. The patient's oxygenation, ventilation, circulation, and temperature should be continuously evaluated. All fluid lines, monitoring cables, and breathing circuits should be long enough to allow safe movement of the angiographic table. Pulse oximetry, placed on the great toe of the leg that will receive the femoral introducer sheath, can qualitatively assess oxygenation and provide early warning of femoral artery occlusion or thrombus. Continuous EKG and blood pressure measurement at least every 3 minutes can detect arrhythmias and any decreases in perfusion. [9] Placement of intra-arterial catheter for continuous blood pressure monitoring is helpful but should not delay endovascular treatment. The side port on the femoral artery introducer sheath can also be used to continuously measure the patient's blood pressure. This method will underestimate systolic and overestimate diastolic pressures due to the catheter within the sheath, but the mean arterial pressures will be accurate.

9.4 Fluid Management

Isotonic crystalloid solutions are recommended for AIS. Patients with chronic hypertension are often volume contracted. This relative hypovolemic state makes these patients prone to hypotension under general anesthesia. Euvolemia should be the therapeutic goal. Hemodilution and hypervolemia has not shown benefit in ischemic stroke.[10] Hypotonic solution such as lactated ringers should be avoided due to increased risk of cerebral edema. Colloids, particularly albumin, have been proposed as being neuroprotective. However, human trials of albumin in acute stroke have shown no neurologic improvement and increased rates of intracerebral hemorrhage and pulmonary edema. [11] Dextrose-containing fluids should be avoided unless the patient is hypoglycemic.

9.5 Temperature

In animal models, mild hypothermia (33–34 °C) has been proven to be effective in reducing the brain's vulnerability to ischemic injury. In humans, clinical trials for aneurysm surgery and head-injured patients failed to show benefit for induced hypothermia. However, hypothermia has been shown to improve neurologic outcomes following cardiac arrest.[12] There is yet to be a large randomized clinical trial studying hypothermia in the setting of ischemic stroke.[13] What is well established however, is that even mild increases in temperature dramatically worsen ischemic brain injury. Therefore, normothermia should be maintained between 35 and 37 °C during endovascular treatment. Patients should be treated with antipyretics and cooling blankets if febrile. Shivering should be treated with meperidine.

9.6 Blood Glucose

Hyperglycemia is an independent risk factor for poor clinical outcomes in ischemic stroke. Hyperglycemia worsens acidosis in the ischemic penumbra through anaerobic glucose metabolism and lactic acid production. Blood glucose level of > 140 mg/dL have been associated with increased mortality and complications, such as intracerebral hemorrhage, in stroke patients receiving thrombolytic therapy.[14] However, intensive insulin therapy is not without risks. Hypoglycemia can worsen brain injury. It can be difficult to safely administer intensive insulin therapy in the setting of endovascular stroke treatment, as patients are transported between different critical care units and multiple providers. Nevertheless, insulin treatment for hyperglycemia should be initiated for blood glucose levels greater than 140 mg/dL. Blood glucose levels below 50 mg/dL should be treated with dextrose infusion for a target blood glucose level greater than 70 mg/dL.[5]

9.7 Arterial Carbon Dioxide and Oxygen Tension

Manipulation of arterial carbon dioxide (CO_2) tension is an effective means of altering cerebral physiology. Hyperventilation and hypocapnia will rapidly decrease cerebral blood flow, cerebral blood volume, and intracranial pressure. Hypocapnia has been shown to worsen ischemic and traumatic brain injury. Hypercapnia will have the opposite, increased effect, on cerebral blood flow and intracranial pressure.[15] There are no clinical studies supporting hypercapnia in ischemic stroke. Normocapnia should be the goal for these patients.

Acute stroke patients are at risk for hypoxia due to stroke symptomatology. Respiratory drive may be impaired as well as the ability to clear secretions and protect the airway. Hyperoxia has been suggested as a neuroprotective therapy and a method to increase the therapeutic time window for revascularization. However, hyperbaric oxygen therapy has failed to improve ischemic stroke outcomes in multiple clinical trials. Supplemental oxygen is indicated during sedation of the stroke patient.[16] Continuous pulse oximetry should be used, with a target SpO2 of greater than 92%. In patients whom oxygenation and ventilation are inadequate, tracheal intubation and mechanical ventilation are indicated until their condition improves.

9.8 Intraprocedural Complications

Complications during endovascular treatment of thromboembolic stroke are rare events that must be recognized early and treated rapidly to minimize injury to the patient. The most serious complications are vessel perforation and intracerebral hemorrhage. Communication between the anesthesiologist and the neuroendovascular surgeon is critical. The first signs of hemorrhage may be contrast extravasation, abrupt neurologic decline, or bradycardic response to increased intracranial pressure (ICP). If sedation, the case should be converted to a general anesthetic, allowing greater control of the patient's hemodynamics and ventilation. Vessel injury should be repaired endovascularly. The minimum safe blood systolic blood pressure is 140 mm Hg.[17] Relative hypotension increases the risk of worsening cerebral ischemia. A fast-acting, easily titratable antihypertensive such as nicardipine is appropriate. Normocapnia should be maintained. If bleeding continues and the patient has received tissue plasminogen activator (tPA), cryoprecipitate can be given to raise fibrinogen levels. Antifibrinolytics, such as tranexamic acid, can also be given to bind plasminogen and inhibit fibrin degradation. Further resuscitation and treatment ICP may include rapid infusion of mannitol, titration of anesthetic to burst suppression, passive cooling, and placement of an external ventricular drain.[4]

9.9 Hemodynamic Management

Blood pressure management during and after AIS is a controversial subject. The majority of acute ischemic patients present with elevated blood pressures. This is primarily due to underlying baseline hypertension. However, there is also an early hypertensive response to cerebral ischemia which further elevates blood pressures in these patients. Systemic blood pressure rises in an attempt to perfuse ischemic regions of the brain. Within the ischemic penumbra there is maximal arteriole dilation, and autoregulation is impaired as cerebral blood flow becomes directly proportional to blood pressure.[18,19] This hypertensive response slowly resolves over the next 12 to 24 hours following the stroke.

Ischemic stroke patients have a U-shaped mortality pattern in relation to their admission blood pressures.[20] Both low and high blood pressures are associated with worse outcomes.[21] In patients treated with tPA, elevated blood pressures are associated with lower recanalization rates.[22,23] Similarly, in patients treated by mechanical thrombectomy, elevated systolic blood pressures are associated with lower recanalization rates.[24] The exact neuroprotective mechanism blood pressure plays in the ischemic penumbra is not yet clear. It appears that the hypertensive response, which improves perfusion of the collateral circulation, at some point become inversely correlated to favorable reperfusion therapy outcomes.[25] Whether blood pressure is itself an independent predictive factor or an active contributor affecting clot retrieval is unknown.

Currently, the accepted body of thinking is that during the AIS periprocedural period, moderate hypertension is of benefit, providing perfusion to ischemic regions.[26] Systolic blood pressure less than 140 mm Hg have been associated with worse outcome in patients undergoing endovascular treatment of AIS with general anesthesia.[27,28] Induced hypertension is reasonable during AIS treatment with a systolic blood pressure goal > 140. Phenylephrine is a good first line choice. A potent alpha-agonist, phenylephrine causes peripheral vasoconstriction, raising blood pressure with few cardiac side effects. However, blood pressure augmentation must be balanced by the possibility that hypertension may result in cerebral hyperemia and edema formation. (Induced hypertension, especially in the setting of tPA administration, could result in catastrophic hemorrhage. Once given tPA, AIS patient blood pressure goals should be less than 180/105 mm Hg to decrease risk of hemorrhage. Calcium channel blockers such as nicardipine or clevidipine, short-acting dihydropyridines, are the preferred agents. This class of drugs is selective for vascular smooth muscle, with little effect on heart rate or contractility.[29] Once thrombectomy has been achieved, the patient's blood pressure should be brought to below 160 mm Hg systolic to decrease risk of hyperemia and hemorrhage.

9.10 Anesthetic Agents Effects on Neurophysiology

It is important to understand the effects of anesthetic agents on cerebral physiology. While most anesthetics have not been specifically been studied in the setting of AIS, it is prudent for the anesthesiologist and proceduralist to have an understanding of how these drugs affect cerebral vasculature and blood flow and to extrapolate how these changes apply to the setting of cerebral ischemia.

9.11 Volatile Agents

Inhaled volatile anesthetics are the most commonly used drugs to maintain general anesthesia today. Volatiles are commonly used for many neurosurgical procedures, including anesthesia for AIS. They have many unique properties which can be either advantageous or detrimental to a patient's neurophysiology depending on how their properties are tailored to the individual stroke patient.

Modern inhaled anesthetics have more similarities than differences. They are all halogenated derivatives of methyl ethyl ether. They are halogenated partly or entirely with fluorine, which provides greater stability and lowers toxicity. These halogenated volatile anesthetics are liquids at room temperature, they are inexpensive, and they have a low solubility in blood. This low blood solubility allows for rapid onset of action, precise control of concentrations during maintenance of anesthesia, and quick exhalation, allowing for rapid awakening and recovery.

The most commonly inhaled agents are isoflurane, sevoflurane, and desflurane. These three agents are very similar with regard to their central nervous system effects. These agents all decrease cerebral metabolic rate (CMR). This decrease in CMR is dose dependent until isoelectric EEG is achieved. There is evidence that volatile and intravenous anesthetic agents may afford some degree of neuroprotection against mild ischemic injury.[30] However, to date, there are no human trials showing anesthetic neuroprotection during focal ischemia.

Volatile anesthetics all increase cerebral blood flow (CBF) through a direct vasodilatory effect. This vasodilation occurs at different concentrations for each individual agent. Generally, though,

in concentrations above 0.6 minimum alveolar concentration (alveolar concentration that prevents movement in 50% of patients), volatile anesthetics will produce a cerebral vasodilation with a resulting dose-dependent increase in CBF.[31] Isoflurane and desflurane have similar CBF increases, with less of an effect seen by sevoflurane. It is important to note that increases in CBF by volatile anesthetics can be attenuated by hypocapnia. Inhaled anesthetics do not affect carbon dioxide cerebral vascular reactivity.[32] Consequently, changes in partial pressure of carbon dioxide between 20 and 80 mm Hg produce changes in CBF. There is a linear change in CBF of 1 to 2 ml/100 g/min per 1 mm Hg increase in partial pressure of CO_2.[33]

Another key difference among the volatile agents is their effect of cerebral autoregulation. Cerebral autoregulation preserves CBF in the face of changing cerebral perfusion pressures (CPP). Normally, CBF is maintained at a constant 50 ml/100 g/min between CPP of 50 to 150 mm Hg. In chronic hypertensive patients, this range is shifted toward higher pressures. The acute stroke patient is likely to have baseline hypertension superimposed upon an early hypertensive response to ischemia. Therefore, the safe lower limit for CPP in these patients is also shifted to the right. Maintaining this higher baseline blood pressure is important during volatile anesthesia because these anesthetics impair autoregulation in a dose-dependent manner. Isoflurane and desflurane impair autoregulation at concentrations greater than 0.5 minimum alveolar concentration (MAC). Sevoflurane retains intact cerebral autoregulation up to 1.5 MAC.[34]

Understanding the inhaled anesthetics interactions and effects on CBF, CO_2 reactivity, and cerebral vascular resistance is critical in the setting of acute stroke. This is because cerebral ischemia causes a disruption in autoregulation, particularly in the ischemic penumbra. In this area, autoregulation and CO_2 reactivity are nearly abolished. Perfusion is passively dependent on cerebral perfusion pressures.[35] Therefore, very precise blood pressure control and respiratory management is needed. A concern in these patients, particularly with the use of volatile anesthesia, is intracerebral steal. This "steal" phenomenon occurs during hypercapnia and volatile anesthesia, causing a shunting of blood away from ischemic areas to those with normal vasoreactivity. Conversely, reverse intracerebral steal or "Robin Hood effect" is theorized to occur when hypocapnia causes an increase in cerebral vascular resistance in normal tissue, therefore shunting blood to ischemic regions.[36] Currently however, there is not enough evidence to recommend either hypocapnia or hypercapnia to alter CBF during stroke. Normocapnia and maintenance of adequate perfusion pressure should be the primary goal.

9.12 Intravenous Agents

The two most commonly used intravenous agents for induction and maintenance of anesthesia in the stroke patient are propofol and barbiturates. Both of these drugs share many similar anesthetic and neurophysiological effects. They both enhance transmission of the inhibitory neurotransmitter gamma-aminobutyric acid (GABA). However, the most common barbiturate, thiopental, is no longer readily available in the United States. Both propofol and thiopental are cerebral vasoconstrictors. They cause both a decrease in CBF and intracranial pressure (ICP). The drop in ICP exceeds the decrease in blood pressure such that that cerebral perfusion pressure is increased. Any decrease in CBF by these agents is offset by a greater decrease in CMR. Both barbiturates and propofol have been shown in animal models to provide brain protection during mild episodes of focal ischemia.[37] But, like the volatile agents, propofol and barbiturate neuroprotection has not been shown with moderate to severe ischemic insults.

9.13 Muscle Relaxants

Modern nondepolarizing muscle relaxants have minimal effects on cerebral physiology. Histamine release and hypotension were a concern with older drugs. Succinylcholine, a fast-acting depolarizing muscle relaxant, has been associated with no or minimal increase in CBF and ICP.[38] However, advantages of its rapid onset of action for full stomach patients far outweigh any risks.

9.14 Anesthesia Adjuncts

Anesthesia adjuncts are medications that can be used to decrease total amount of general anesthetic used. They also can be administered alone for conscious sedation, avoiding general anesthesia altogether. Midazolam and fentanyl are most commonly used for sedation. They are titratable, reversible, and administered routinely by nonanesthesia providers. Midazolam, a short acting benzodiazepine, acts on GABA receptors. Midazolam modestly decreases CBF and CMR and increases the seizure threshold. Disadvantages of midazolam in the AIS patient are an increased risk of delirium and respiratory depression. Fentanyl, a short-acting synthetic opioid, may also cause respiratory depression and can make neurologic assessment difficult. Dexmedetomidine, an alpha-2 adrenergic agonist, is an adjunct with a favorable cerebral physiological profile. As a clonidine analogue, its main advantage is sedation without respiratory depression.[39] Dexmedetomidine is known to provide cooperative sedation with a lower incidence of postoperative delirium and agitation compared to other agents.[40] These attributes make dexmedetomidine an excellent choice for sedation during AIS therapy.

9.15 Anesthetic Technique for Acute Ischemic Stroke Therapy

The optimal anesthetic for AIS therapy remains a point of contention. Members of major neurointerventional societies have been evenly split between general anesthesia versus sedation for AIS.[41] Many proceduralists and anesthesiologists feel that general anesthesia affords a greater degree of safety. Advantages of general anesthesia are a motionless patient, a protected airway, and controlled ventilation.[42] Advantages of sedation include intraprocedural neurologic evaluation and smoother hemodynamics. Some experts feel that induction of a general anesthetic not only delays the start of the procedure, but also causes disruptions to blood pressure and neurophysiology, potentially magnifying cerebral insult and injury.[43]

Nearly all large, retrospective studies comparing conscious sedation to general anesthesia in AIS therapy have shown worse outcomes in patients undergoing general anesthesia.[44,45,46] Specifically, the degree of revascularization and patient disability following thrombectomy was significantly worse in general anesthesia patients.[47] These patients had higher mortality, longer length of stay, increased hospital cost, and higher rates of pneumonia and tracheostomy.[48,49] Compared to sedation, induction of general anesthesia has been associated with concomitant hypotension and worsening neurologic outcomes.[27] General anesthesia has also been correlated with delays in time to treatment.[50] However, all of these studies are limited by their retrospective design. Selection bias likely influenced conclusion validity, as general anesthesia patients tended to be sicker, with significantly higher admission NIHSS scores.

Recently there have been prospective randomized controlled trials evaluating sedation versus general anesthesia for endovascular treatment in AIS. In the Sedation vs. Intubation for Endovascular Stroke Treatment (SIESTA) trial, patients selected for thrombectomy were randomized to receive either general anesthesia or sedation. There was no difference in early neurologic improvement in NIHSS after 24 hours and no differences in mortality between the two groups.[51] The Anesthesia During Stroke (AnStroke) study also found no difference between general anesthesia and conscious sedation in neurologic outcome 3 months after stroke.[52] In both of these studies, there were no differences in hemodynamics between the two groups. The AnStroke trial went as far to set strict systolic blood pressure goals of 140 to 160 mm Hg.

Minimal or no sedation is the anesthetic of choice at our institution. Numerous retrospective studies showing worse outcomes with general anesthesia and our early adoption of the direct aspiration first pass technique (ADAPT) for thrombectomy guided our decision to use conscious sedation.[53] The ADAPT technique involves direct first-pass thrombus aspiration through a large bore catheter alone to achieve reperfusion. Adjunctive therapy, such as retrieval devices, is only used when needed. This technique has faster procedural times, which facilitate patient cooperation for conscious sedation.[54] Strict hemodynamic parameters are also maintained during endovascular treatment. Intraprocedure systolic blood pressures goals are 140 to 180 mm Hg, and postprocedure systolic blood pressure should be less than 140 mm Hg.

Recent studies showing equivocal outcomes for general anesthesia and conscious sedation in endovascular stroke treatment raise the point that perhaps the type of anesthetic is less important than the experience of the anesthesia provider. An experienced and appropriately trained anesthesia team is vital for patient care. The optimal anesthetic for AIS is one where physiological goals are understood and quickly achieved to minimize cerebral insult to the patient.

References

[1] Newton MC. Anaesthesia for Neuroimaging and Interventional Neuroradiology. Anaesth Intensive Care Med. 2007; 8 (10):423–426

[2] Young WL, Pile-Spellman J. Anesthetic considerations for interventional neuroradiology. Anesthesiology. 1994; 80(2): 427–456

[3] Metzner J, Posner KL, Domino KB. The risk and safety of anesthesia at remote locations: the US closed claims analysis. Curr Opin Anaesthesiol. 2009; 22(4):502–508

[4] Jauch EC, Saver JL, Adams HP, Jr, et al. American Heart Association Stroke Council, Council on Cardiovascular Nursing, Council on Peripheral Vascular Disease, Council on Clinical Cardiology. Guidelines for the early management of patients with acute ischemic stroke: a guideline for healthcare professionals from the American Heart Association/American Stroke Association. Stroke. 2013; 44(3):870–947

[5] Talke PO, Sharma D, Heyer EJ, Bergese SD, Blackham KA, Stevens RD. Republished: Society for Neuroscience in Anesthesiology and Critical Care expert consensus statement: Anesthetic management of endovascular treatment for acute ischemic stroke. Stroke. 2014; 45(8):e138–e150

[6] el-Ganzouri AR, McCarthy RJ, Tuman KJ, Tanck EN, Ivankovich AD. Preoperative airway assessment: predictive value of a multivariate risk index. Anesth Analg. 1996; 82(6):1197–1204

[7] Kheterpal S, Martin L, Shanks AM, Tremper KK. Prediction and outcomes of impossible mask ventilation: a review of 50,000 anesthetics. Anesthesiology. 2009; 110(4):891–897

[8] Rose DK, Cohen MM. The airway: problems and predictions in 18,500 patients. Can J Anaesth. 1994; 41(5 Pt 1):372–383

[9] Lee CZ, Litt L, Hashimoto T, Young WL. Physiologic monitoring and anesthesia considerations in acute ischemic stroke. J Vasc Interv Radiol. 2004; 15(1 Pt 2):S13–S19

[10] Chang TS, Jensen MB. Hemodilution for acute ischemic stroke. Stroke. 2015; 46(1):e4–e5

[11] Martin RH, Yeatts SD, Hill MD, Moy CS, Ginsberg MD, Palesch YY, ALIAS Parts 1 and 2 and NETT Investigators. ALIAS (Albumin in Acute Ischemic Stroke) Trials: Analysis of the Combined Data From Parts 1 and 2. Stroke. 2016; 47(9): 2355–2359

[12] Hypothermia after Cardiac Arrest Study Group. Mild therapeutic hypothermia to improve the neurologic outcome after cardiac arrest. N Engl J Med. 2002; 346(8):549–556

[13] Wu TC, Grotta JC. Hypothermia for acute ischaemic stroke. Lancet Neurol. 2013; 12(3):275–284

[14] Alvarez-Sabín J, Molina CA, Montaner J, et al. Effects of admission hyperglycemia on stroke outcome in reperfused tissue plasminogen activator–treated patients. Stroke. 2003; 34(5):1235–1241

[15] Messick JM, Jr, Newberg LA, Nugent M, Faust RJ. Principles of neuroanesthesia for the nonneurosurgical patient with CNS pathophysiology. Anesth Analg. 1985; 64(2):143–174

[16] Singhal AB. A review of oxygen therapy in ischemic stroke. Neurol Res. 2007; 29(2):173–183

[17] Frontera JA, Lewin JJ, III, Rabinstein AA, et al. Guideline for Reversal of Antithrombotics in Intracranial Hemorrhage: A Statement for Healthcare Professionals from the Neurocritical Care Society and Society of Critical Care Medicine. Neurocrit Care. 2016; 24(1):6–46

[18] Goldstein LB. Blood pressure management in patients with acute ischemic stroke. Hypertension. 2004; 43(2):137–141

[19] Meyer JS, Shimazu K, Fukuuchi Y, Ouchi T, Okamoto S, Koto A. Impaired neurogenic cerebrovascular control and dysautoregulation after stroke. Stroke. 1973; 4(2):169–186

[20] Leonardi-Bee J, Bath PM, Phillips SJ, Sandercock PA, IST Collaborative Group. Blood pressure and clinical outcomes in the International Stroke Trial. Stroke. 2002; 33(5):1315–1320

[21] Vemmos KN, Tsivgoulis G, Spengos K, et al. U-shaped relationship between mortality and admission blood pressure in patients with acute stroke. J Intern Med. 2004; 255 (2):257–265

[22] Huang Y, Sharma VK, Robinson T, et al. ENCHANTED investigators. Rationale, design, and progress of the ENhanced Control of Hypertension ANd Thrombolysis strokE stuDy (ENCHANTED) trial: An international multicenter 2 × 2 quasi-factorial randomized controlled trial of low- vs. standard-dose rt-PA and early intensive vs. guideline-recommended blood pressure lowering in patients with acute ischaemic stroke eligible for thrombolysis treatment. Int J Stroke. 2015; 10(5):778–788

[23] Tsivgoulis G, Saqqur M, Sharma VK, Lao AY, Hill MD, Alexandrov AV, CLOTBUST Investigators. Association of pretreatment blood pressure with tissue plasminogen activator-induced arterial recanalization in acute ischemic stroke. Stroke. 2007; 38(3):961–966

[24] Nogueira RG, Liebeskind DS, Sung G, Duckwiler G, Smith WS, MERCI, Multi MERCI Writing Committee. Predictors of good clinical outcomes, mortality, and successful revascularization in patients with acute ischemic stroke undergoing thrombectomy: pooled analysis of the Mechanical Embolus Removal in Cerebral Ischemia (MERCI) and Multi MERCI Trials. Stroke. 2009; 40(12):3777–3783

[25] Regenhardt RW, Das AS, Stapleton CJ, et al. Blood Pressure and Penumbral Sustenance in Stroke from Large Vessel Occlusion. Front Neurol. 2017; 8:317

[26] Mistri AK, Robinson TG, Potter JF. Pressor therapy in acute ischemic stroke: systematic review. Stroke. 2006; 37(6):1565–1571

[27] Davis MJ, Menon BK, Baghirzada LB, et al. Calgary Stroke Program. Anesthetic management and outcome in patients during endovascular therapy for acute stroke. Anesthesiology. 2012; 116(2):396–405

[28] Treurniet KM, et al. A Decrease in Blood Pressure Is Associated with Unfavorable Outcome in Patients Undergoing Thrombectomy under General Anesthesia. J Neurointerv Surg. 2017; •••:12988

[29] Appleton JP, et al. "Blood Pressure Management in Acute Stroke." Stroke and Vascular Neurology. BMJ Specialist Journals. 2016; 1(2):72–82

[30] Warner DS, Zhou JG, Ramani R, Todd MM. Reversible focal ischemia in the rat: effects of halothane, isoflurane, and methohexital anesthesia. J Cereb Blood Flow Metab. 1991; 11 (5):794–802

[31] Matta BF, Heath KJ, Tipping K, Summors AC. Direct cerebral vasodilatory effects of sevoflurane and isoflurane. Anesthesiology. 1999; 91(3):677–680

[32] Strebel S, Kaufmann M, Baggi M, Zenklusen U. Cerebrovascular carbon dioxide reactivity during exposure to equipotent isoflurane and isoflurane in nitrous oxide anaesthesia. Br J Anaesth. 1993; 71(2):272–276

[33] Kuroda Y, Murakami M, Tsuruta J, Murakawa T, Sakabe T. Blood flow velocity of middle cerebral artery during prolonged anesthesia with halothane, isoflurane, and sevoflurane in humans. Anesthesiology. 1997; 87(3):527–532

[34] Summors AC, Gupta AK, Matta BF. Dynamic cerebral autoregulation during sevoflurane anesthesia: a comparison with isoflurane. Anesth Analg. 1999; 88(2):341–345

[35] Aries MJH, Elting JW, De Keyser J, Kremer BP, Vroomen PC. Cerebral autoregulation in stroke: a review of transcranial Doppler studies. Stroke. 2010; 41(11):2697–2704

[36] Lassen NA, Christensen MS. Physiology of cerebral blood flow. Br J Anaesth. 1976; 48(8):719–734

[37] Kochs E, Hoffman WE, Werner C, Thomas C, Albrecht RF, Schulte am Esch J. The effects of propofol on brain electrical activity, neurologic outcome, and neuronal damage following incomplete ischemia in rats. Anesthesiology. 1992; 76(2):245–252

[38] Kovarik W D, Mayberg TS, Lam AM, et al. "Succinylcholine Does Not Change Intracranial Pressure, Cerebral Blood Flow Velocity, or the Electroencephalogram in Patients with Neurologic Injury.". Anesthesia & Analgesia. 1994; 78(3):469–473

[39] Drummond JC, Dao AV, Roth DM, et al. Effect of dexmedetomidine on cerebral blood flow velocity, cerebral metabolic rate, and carbon dioxide response in normal humans. Anesthesiology. 2008; 108(2):225–232

[40] Wang X, Ji J, Fen L, Wang A. Effects of dexmedetomidine on cerebral blood flow in critically ill patients with or without traumatic brain injury: a prospective controlled trial. Brain Inj. 2013; 27(13–14):1617–1622

[41] Mehta B, Leslie-Mazwi TM, Chandra RV, et al. Assessing variability in neurointerventional practice patterns for acute ischemic stroke. J Neurointerv Surg. 2013; 5 Suppl 1:i52–i57

[42] Brekenfeld C, Mattle HP, Schroth G. General is better than local anesthesia during endovascular procedures. Stroke. 2010; 41(11):2716–2717

[43] Anastasian ZH. Anaesthetic management of the patient with acute ischaemic stroke. Br J Anaesth. 2014; 113 Suppl 2:ii9–ii16

[44] Bekelis K, Missios S, MacKenzie TA, Tjoumakaris S, Jabbour P. Anesthesia Technique and Outcomes of Mechanical Thrombectomy in Patients With Acute Ischemic Stroke. Stroke. 2017; 48(2):361–366

[45] Berkhemer OA, van den Berg LA, Fransen PS, et al. MR CLEAN investigators. The effect of anesthetic management during intra-arterial treatment for acute stroke in MR CLEAN. Neurology. 2016; 87(7):656–664

[46] Brinjikji W, Murad MH, Rabinstein AA, Cloft HJ, Lanzino G, Kallmes DF. Conscious sedation versus general anesthesia during endovascular acute ischemic stroke treatment: a systematic review and meta-analysis. AJNR Am J Neuroradiol. 2015; 36(3):525–529

[47] Abou-Chebl A, Yeatts SD, Yan B, et al. Impact of General Anesthesia on Safety and Outcomes in the Endovascular Arm of Interventional Management of Stroke (IMS) III Trial. Stroke. 2015; 46(8):2142–2148

[48] Jumaa MA, Zhang F, Ruiz-Ares G, et al. Comparison of safety and clinical and radiographic outcomes in endovascular acute stroke therapy for proximal middle cerebral artery occlusion with intubation and general anesthesia versus the nonintubated state. Stroke. 2010; 41(6):1180–1184

[49] McDonald JS, Brinjikji W, Rabinstein AA, Cloft HJ, Lanzino G, Kallmes DF. Conscious sedation versus general anaesthesia during mechanical thrombectomy for stroke: a propensity score analysis. J Neurointerv Surg. 2015; 7(11):789–794

[50] van den Berg LA, Koelman DL, Berkhemer OA, et al. MR CLEAN pretrial study group, Participating centers. Type of anesthesia and differences in clinical outcome after intra-arterial treatment for ischemic stroke. Stroke. 2015; 46(5):1257–1262

[51] Schönenberger S, Uhlmann L, Hacke W, et al. Effect of Conscious Sedation vs General Anesthesia on Early Neurological Improvement Among Patients With Ischemic Stroke Undergoing Endovascular Thrombectomy: A Randomized Clinical Trial. JAMA. 2016; 316(19):1986–1996

[52] Löwhagen Hendén P, Rentzos A, Karlsson JE, et al. General Anesthesia Versus Conscious Sedation for Endovascular Treatment of Acute Ischemic Stroke: The AnStroke Trial (Anesthesia During Stroke). Stroke. 2017; 48(6):1601–1607

[53] Turk AS, Frei D, Fiorella D, et al. ADAPT FAST study: a direct aspiration first pass technique for acute stroke thrombectomy. J Neurointerv Surg. 2014; 6(4):260–264

[54] Turk AS, Spiotta A, Frei D, et al. Initial clinical experience with the ADAPT technique: a direct aspiration first pass technique for stroke thrombectomy. J Neurointerv Surg. 2014; 6(3):231–237

10 Neurocritical Care of the Acute Ischemic Stroke

Ana Canale, Pedro Grille, and Paul Vespa

Abstract

Acute stroke remains one of the leading causes of mortality and disability worldwide. Ischemic stroke represents approximately 80% of all types of strokes.

In the last twenty years, the acute management of stroke have change dramatically. The development of the Strokes Center, Stroke Unit and the Reperfusion therapy with intravenous tissue plasminogen activator (IV rTPA) and/or endovascular thrombectomy, all have contributed to improve outcomes. Even though, still remain up to 20% of patients with the most severely acute ischemic stroke (AIS) who will benefit from specialized neurocritical care (NCC).

The objective of this chapter is to review the management of AIS patients focusing in clinical and evidence based aspects.

The intensive care management for severely AIS must be developed by a multidisciplinary team and aggressively and meticulous supportive care is essential to ensure optimal neurologic outcomes.

Through intensive monitoring and specialized treatment, the main goals are: early recognition of neuroworsening prioritizing non-invasive neuromonitoring, reducing complications of reperfusion, such as hemorrhagic transformation, and minimizing secondary brain injury, including brain edema and progressive stroke. Critical issues that might modulate neurological outcome include blood pressure and glucose optimization, avoidance of fever, fluid and nutritional management, early rehabilitation and the management of medical complications and comorbidities.

Keywords: ischemic stroke, neurocritical care, neuroworsening, cerebral infarct

10.1 Introduction

Despite of the advances in the diagnosis and treatment of acute stroke, it remains one of the leading causes of mortality and disability in the developed world. Ischemic stroke represents approximately 80% of all types of strokes. In the last two decades the acute management of stroke patients has evolved to stroke unit and stroke centers with improved outcomes, including reduced in-hospital length of stay and decreased mortality.[1] Up to 20% of these patients benefit from neurocritical care.[2] Several studies have demonstrated the beneficial effect of specialized neurocritical care (NCC) team intervention in these patients.[3]

The critical care of the Acute Ischemic Stroke (AIS) patients must be developed by a multidisciplinary team, and is based on vital support, early recognition of neuroworsening, optimizing cerebral perfusion, minimizing the reperfusion injury, and finally avoid and treat neurologic and systemic complications.[4]

In this chapter, we will review the clinical aspects of critical care of AIS patients, with emphasis in a practical and evidence based approach.

10.2 Indications for Admission to the Intensive Care Unit

Patients suffering an AIS require NCC due to several situations.[5,6] Although there is variability in the criteria for intensive care unit (ICU) admission, the following indications are accepted for the majority of the authors (► Table 10.1):

a) Severe neurological deficits with the need of artificial airway and mechanical ventilation due to depressed level of consciousness or reduced ability to protect their airway,

b) Risk of neurological worsening, like: severe stroke score (NIHSS > 17), large hemispheric infarcts (> 145 cc), significant infarcts involving the brainstem or cerebellum, significant mass effect or brain shift in the computed tomography.

c) Need to specialized non-invasive or invasive neurologic monitoring or specific therapy for intracranial hypertension or cerebral edema.

d) Generalized seizures or status epilepticus.

e) Post-surgical interventions: decompressive craniectomy, evacuation of cerebellar infarct or ventriculostomy for hydrocephalus in posterior fossa infarcts.

f) Patients with significant cardiovascular, respiratory or systemic dysfunction due to comorbidities or complications: pulmonary edema or embolism, acute heart failure, hypotension that requires vasopressors, severe arterial hypertension with the need of intravenous medications, arrhythmias, aortic

Table 10.1 Indications for ICU admission in AIS patients

Severe neurological deficit	• Need for endotracheal intubation and mechanical ventilation
Risk of neuroworsening	• NIHSS > 17 • Large hemispheric infarcts (> 145 cc) • Significant infarcts involving the brainstem or cerebellum • Significant mass effect or brain shift in the CT.
Generalized seizure or status epilepticus	• Specific treatment for cerebral edema
Post-surgical interventions:	• Decompressive craniectomy • Evacuation of cerebellar infarct • Ventriculostomy for hydrocephalus in posterior fossa infarcts
Significant comorbidities or complications that may need specific monitorization	• Pulmonary edema or embolism • Acute heart failure • Hypotension that requires vasopressors • Uncontrolled hypertension • Arrhythmias • Aortic dissection • Metabolic abnormalities that require specific • close monitoring

dissection or metabolic abnormalities that require specific close monitoring.

g) Immediate Post-thrombolysis or post-thrombectomy for hemodynamic and neurologic monitoring.

In these group of patients, as it was previously mentioned, specialized NCC units have shown to improve outcomes and decrease their length of stay.[7,8] Another important topic of these patients is that delay in their admission to an ICU was significantly associated with a worse outcome, so they should be admitted as soon as possible.[9]

10.3 Neuroworsening: Detection of Neurological Deterioration

Neurological deterioration or neuroworsening constitutes a cornerstone in the management of patients suffering AIS. Neurological examination is the most important tool to detect it, since intracranial pressure (ICP) monitoring, have limitations in

detect and predict neurological deterioration after ischemic stroke.[10,11] Neuroworsening after stroke commonly is due to one four mechanisms: 1) Brain edema with tissue shift, which does not necessarily cause elevated ICP but can cause an herniation syndrome, 2) Hemorrhagic transformation with worsening of mass effect and potentially elevated ICP, 3) Collateral cerebral blood flow failure with extension of the ischemic brain, and 4) seizures which can elicit a reduction in the level of consciousness with or without worsening brain edema and tissue shift.

The National Institutes of Health Stroke Scale (NHISS) is the most common standardized and efficient score used to evaluate the clinical status of AIS. An increase of two or more points is considered a threshold for significant neuroworsening. In patients with severe consciousness compromise, the specifically designed Glasgow Coma Scale (GCS) may be more useful.[5,12] Additional score that is useful for neurological monitoring is the Full Outline of Unresponsiveness Score (FOUR Score), which permits a detailed assessment of language, motor, brainstem and breathing functions. The use of the FOUR score is now recommended for patients with stupor and/or coma.

The evaluation of pupillary size and reactivity to light is a fundamental part of the neurological examination, which is crucial in patients who are deteriorating due to cerebral midline shift or transtentorial herniation. The utilization of the infrared pupillometry, provide a non-invasive and bedside method, which eliminates limitations of the manual way of pupillary clinical assessment, like subjectivity, inconsistency and highly interobserver variability. We use the portable infrared pupilometer (Forsite NeurOptics, Irvine, CA ®), which allows an automated, accurate, easy, quick, reproducible and quantitative measure of different pupillary parameters including: maximum and minimum apertures, percentage of aperture change following light stimulation, constriction and dilation velocities, and latency period[13,14]

Routine ICP monitoring is not recommended in AIS, because significant tissue and brain herniation may occur in the absence of elevated ICP. Hence intracranial hypertension is a late sign of neuroworsening and ICP values are often normal even in the presence of large ischemic tissue volume. There are no randomized clinical trials evaluating ICP monitoring in stroke patients.[3,15]

In a prospective study, Poca et al found that the majority of patients with malignant middle cerebral artery infarct had ICP values less than

20 mmHg. In this study, pupillary abnormalities, cerebral midline shift and brainstem compression were present despite normal ICP values.[11] The relative value of ICP monitoring in predicting neuro-worsening could be explained because the stroke is a focal lesion, and the compartmentalized ICP phenomenon may not reflect the pressure in the contralateral hemisphere or infratentorium. Other hypothesis could be that the distance between the ICP probe site and the brain herniation site, in generally the tentorial notch, is inversely proportional to the pressure gradient force. This is very important because we know now that there are morphometric anatomic variations of the structure of the tentorial notch, which could explain why some patients who have a narrow subtype of tentorial notch deteriorates earlier than others who have a large one.[16] We have recently developed a computed tomographic protocol to measure the tentorial notch, so we could be able to predict which stroke patient are at risk of neuroworsening based on their morphometric anatomic variation of tentorial notch (preliminary data, not shown).

Having said this, there is a place for the use of ventriculostomy for the treatment of obstructive hydrocephalus complicating cerebellar stroke, subarachnoid hemorrhage, cerebellar hemorrhage, and primary intraparenchymal hemorrhage (ICH). Ventriculostomy use to drain cerebrospinal fluid and relieve hydrocephalus is a treatment option in these conditions. However, posterior fossa brain edema from cerebellar stroke is best treated by surgical craniectomy and decompression rather than by ventriculostomy alone.

Invasive multimodal monitoring, including ptO2 or cerebral microdialysis, have not been sufficiently studied in AIS patients, so the routine use of them cannot be recommended at present.[3]

Noninvasive methods of neuromonitoring are becoming a complimentary tool to clinical examination and to predict malignant course of AIS patients:

1. *Ultrasound*: Measure of the optic nerve sheath diameter (ONSD) is an accurate, simple and rapid method for detecting ICP immediate changes and elevated.[17] Recently, it was described a reliable assessment of cerebral midline shift by transcranial color-coded duplex. It has the advantage of bedside available and favorable safety profile, especially in unstable patients in whom performing serial CT scans expose.[18]

2. *Continuous Electroencephalography* (cEEG) monitoring. There are limiting data regarding the utility of the cEEG monitoring in predict or manage AIS patients. Resent studies using continuous and quantitative EEG monitoring in ischemic stroke patients, showed a good correlation between loss of fast EEG activity and low CPP, and between brain symmetry index and NIHSS. This could be a promising non-invasive monitoring technique to estimate or predict the outcome after AIS.[19,20]

10.4 Airway Management and Mechanical Ventilation

Management of the airway is the first step of the medical support of any severe brain injured patient. It is part of the initial triad A, B, C algorithm: airway, breathing and circulation.

Endotracheal intubation is indicated in patients with: a) Decreased level of consciousness; b) Inability to airway protection due to brainstem dysfunction; c) Signs of intracranial hypertension or very large infarcts; d) Any respiratory failure that requires mechanical ventilation.

There are no evidence-based guidelines for specific indication or timing for intubation in AIS. Although, GCS score < 9 is taken as a limit to intubate the decision must be guided by global clinical judgment. In this sense, patients that cannot follow commands due to decreased level of consciousness are candidates to endotracheal intubation, independently of the GCS score.[3,6,10] Intubation within the first 48 hs in large territory ischemic strokes and with low GCS would be reasonable, since that is the window of neuroworsening.

The different guidelines recommend providing *supplemental oxygen* to keep the oxygen saturation level above 94%. Routine supplemental oxygen for all stroke patients or hyperoxia have not demonstrated a significant benefit in randomized clinical studies.[21,22,23]

Hyperventilation should only be used for short periods of time as a rescue therapeutic intervention to reduce ICP in AIS patients with significant cerebral edema and clinical signs of brain herniation. Due to worsening ischemic injury from vasoconstriction, which elicits further ischemia, prophylactic or routine hyperventilation did not demonstrate benefit of outcome in these patients and is not recommended.[3,24]

Respiratory insufficiency occurs in approximately 10 – 20% of AIS patients. There are several causes for it: central hypoventilation due to brainstem infarctions, aspiration pneumonitis or pneumonia, acute lung injury or acute respiratory distress syndrome, cardiogenic or neurogenic pulmonary edema, pulmonary embolism, or respiratory muscle weakness.[2,4]

Noninvasive ventilation should not be used in these patients, because it does not correct underlying problems that frequently present in AIS patients such as central hypoventilation and inability of airway protection due to brainstem dysfunction.

Weaning mechanical ventilation in a severe stroke patient is fundamentally different than the typical non-neurologic ICU patient with respiratory failure. The typical weaning parameters of vital capacity, negative inspiratory force, maximal expiratory force, spontaneous breathing trials, etc do not measure airway control. Airway control and airway protective reflexes are often impaired in severe acute ischemic stroke. While spontaneous breathing trials (SBTs) can be safely done in some patients, SBTs should be avoided in stroke patients with critical brain edema. Gradual weaning of the ventilator rate may be a more cautious approach.

There are some criteria to consider in AIS patients prior to extubation: follow more than one command, successful of spontaneous breathing test, absence of oro-pharyngeal saliva collections, and adequate cough effort measured by the white card test.[25,26]

Tracheostomy should be considered in AIS patients who failed extubation or in whom this is not possible by 7–10 days of mechanical ventilation, typically patients with large MCA or posterior fossa infarcts. The optimal timing for tracheostomy is still matter of debate and is controversial whether early tracheostomy impacts upon AIS patient outcome.[27,28]

In this sense, Schonenberger et al. developed the SET score, which evaluates three areas of assessment: neurological function (dysphagia, observed aspiration and GCS on admission < 10), type and localization of neurological lesion (brainstem, cerebellar or MCA territory), and general organ function (acute lung injury, APACHE II score > 20, sepsis or neurosurgical intervention). They demonstrated in a prospectively study that a SETscore cut-off value of > 8 points predicts prolonged mechanical ventilation and tracheostomy need with a sensitivity of 64% and a specificity of 86%.[29]

Bosel et al. found in a randomized pilot trial of ischemic and hemorrhagic stroke patients, that early tracheostomy group (performed 1–3 days after intubation) had lower ICU mortality (10 vs. 47%) than standard tracheostomy group patients

(7–14 days from intubation).[30] Following this line, the SETPOINT2 is an ongoing multicenter randomized trial in which patients with ischemic or hemorrhagic stroke on mechanical ventilation are randomized to early percutaneous tracheostomy (first five days after intubation) or prolonged orotracheal intubation. This trial might clarify the value of early tracheostomy in these patients.[31]

10.5 Hemodynamic Management

The main objectives of the hemodynamic management of AIS patients are:
a) Avoid hypovolemia and hypotension
b) Hypertension control in certain situations
c) Early recognition and treat cardiac complications.

Basic cardiovascular monitoring includes continuous electrocardiography, noninvasive blood pressure (BP), at least once echocardiography and repeated troponin measures, especially in patients with electrocardiographic or echocardiographic abnormalities.

Patients who are hemodynamic unstable or develop significant cardiac complications, benefit of invasive BP monitoring and might require minimally invasive hemodynamic monitoring such as PiCCO or VIGILANCE ® dispositive, which measure continuous cardiac output, systemic vascular resistances and SvO2.

There is not a specific goal for blood pressure range for AIS patients. Hypovolemia and hypotension must be avoided because they could exacerbate brain ischemia, especially in chronic hypertensive patients in which the autoregulation curve shifts to the right. A mean arterial pressure (MAP) > 85 mmHg appears a reasonable goal in ischemic stroke without hemorrhagic transformation.

Fluid balance should be carefully monitored and managed to achieve euvolemia. Fluid resuscitation with isotonic saline solutions (NaCl 0.9%) is the first step of this management, following by vasoactive agents such as norepinephrine if hypotension is unresponsive to volume replacement. Cautious use of balanced crystalloid solutions may be option but avoidance of hyponatremia is paramount in considering fluid selection.

Almost 80% of total AIS patients are hypertensive upon arrival at the hospital emergency and generally normalize over the first 48 hours. This may be related to several reasons: chronic hypertension, stress, pain or agitation or intracranial hypertension.[32] It was observed a U-shaped relationship between BP and mortality in stroke, with adverse effects on outcome associated to systolic blood pressure (SBP) bellow and above 150 mmHg.[33] BP lowering may exacerbate neurological deterioration by decreasing cerebral perfusion pressure in penumbra tissue when cerebral autoregulation is impaired. On the other hand, severe hypertension can lead to increased brain edema formation and intracerebral hemorrhage due to breakdown of blood-brain barrier, and contribute to cardio-respiratory and renal complications.

This fact, added to the inconsistent evidence of an optimal BP level, makes the management of BP in AIS patients a controversial issue. Clinical guidelines recommend a strategy of permissive hypertension, and BP is allowed to rise as high as 220/120 mm Hg before treatment is started, unless the patient develops cardiac or renal dysfunction due to hypertension (myocardial ischemia, congestive heart or renal failure). In patients who receive intravenous thrombolytic therapy, a strict BP control is needed to keep BP bellow 180/105 mmHg.[3, 10,22] Intravenous labetalol is the agent of choice to lower BP, and nicardipine could be a reasonable option when beta blockers are contraindicated.[34] It must be noted that BP variability in the early phase of ischemic stroke is associated with infarct expansion and worse outcome, so it should be avoided.[35]

There are at least five randomized clinical trials that studied acute BP lowering in nonthrombolyzed ischemic stroke. Two of them (the CHHIPS and COSSACS trial) where small and underpowered, and did not find substantial differences in outcome between treat or placebo groups.[36,37] After, three large randomized clinical trials were developed. The SCAST studied enrolled 2029 patients in nine European countries and found that reducing BP with candesartan in the first 7 days of stroke had no beneficial effects on outcome.[38] The CATIS trial was a randomized studied that enrolled 4071 AIS patients in China, and found no reduction in death or major disability.[39] Finally, the ENOS trial, a partial-factorial randomized study of the effect of transdermal glyceryl trinitrate to lowering BP in the first 7 days of ischemic or hemorrhagic stroke, did not improve outcome in these patients.[40]

Finally, the ENCHANTED trial is an ongoing randomized study to establish the effect of low-dose rtPA and early intensive blood pressure lowering in AIS patients, that might clear out this problem in the next few years[41].

There is no strong evidence for application of induced hypertension in AIS patients.

However, in highly selected patients (with fluctuating or deteriorating neurological status, severely stenotic or occluded major vessel and SBP < 150 mmHg), a strategy of induced hypertension could be carefully applied.[10,42] In this situation, measuring dynamic cerebral autoregulation by transcranial Doppler, like the autoregulation index (ARI) or Mx index, could help to guide hemodynamic management decisions. It is generally accepted that cerebral autoregulation is altered in ischemic and hemorrhagic stroke, and also may change with time and pathological progression. The presence or absence of cerebral autoregulation in acute stroke is critical to maintenance of stable blood flow in the ischemic penumbra and for avoidance of excessive hyperperfusion. It is possible that the subpopulation of AIS patients with relative intact cerebral autoregulation may benefit from aggressive blood pressure treatment to improve clinical outcome.[43] Prospective studies are needed, so today; the practice should be made at individualizing care with the discretion of neurointensivist and neurologist.

There are no specific studies about management of blood pressure in the peri-procedural endovascular setting, such as post mechanical thrombectomy.[44]

In general, the management should be made at individualizing care based on avoiding hypovolemia and hypotension and evaluating the degree of revascularization, the collateral blood flow of ischemic brain tissue and the extent of infarction. For patients with unsuccessful revascularization, the authors recommend permissive hypertension to augment collateralization or even induced hypertension if there is no neurological improvement.

Cardiac complications are common in AIS and explain up to 20% of the mortality after ischemic stroke. Arrhythmias are present in 57% of patients; elevated serum troponin levels in up to 10 to 18%, and 12% have ventricular wall motion abnormalities on echocardiography. Neurogenic stunned myocardium is a cardiac dysfunction seen in various severe intracranial disorders apart from ischemic stroke, cause by catecholamine release, which lead to contraction band necrosis, an described in specific situations as Takotsubo cardiomyopathy. This name is due to its echocardiographic appearance similar to a Japanese vase.[6,45,46,47]

There is no consensus to guide the management of these complications, and the best clinical practice must counterbalance the effects of cardiopulmonary support with the effect of potential neurological worsening. For rapid ventricular rate arrhythmias, beta-blockers and calcium channel blockers are generally used. For hemodynamic instability due to myocardial dysfunction, the therapeutic strategy includes avoidance of fluid overload, supportive care including inotropic drugs and treatment of causal neurologic issues.[10,48,49]

10.6 Cerebral Edema and Intracranial Hypertension Management

The developing of space-occupying edema, which determines progressive neurological deterioration, called malignant cerebral edema, is a life threatening condition in AIS. It occurs in approximately 10% of all ischemic strokes and is associated with an elevated mortality. The main consequences of malignant brain edema are cerebral distortion due to intracranial pressure gradient differences and intracranial hypertension. The common final route of these two phenomena is central or lateral brain herniation. The main cause of intracranial hypertension in AIS is cerebral edema. Other causes are less frequent and required specific treatment such as ventricular drainage of hydrocephalus.

Edema following ischemia and infarction is mediated by various cellular mechanisms: 1) Cytotoxic or ionic edema: the reduced availability of oxygen compromise the energy dependent transport channels of neuron cellular membranes causing loss of ionic gradient and water inflow into neurons, 2) Energy failure of the blood-brain barrier that lead to move fluids into the interstitial space, producing delayed vasogenic edema, 3) Other mechanisms of malignant edema in stroke includes vascular endothelial factors, thrombin and matrix metalloproteinase.[5]

In recent years, it was found the up-regulation of sulfonylurea receptor (Sur-1) regulated channels as another key molecular event involved in the microvascular dysfunction that generate second injury and edema formation, with novel therapeutic implications.[50]

Treatment of malignant cerebral edema includes 2 steps: 1) medical transient management and 2) surgical treatment.

1) *Medical transient management of cerebral edema and intracranial hypertension*:

Stabilization of the airway, breathing and circulation are the first measures for treating intracranial hypertension. Following ABC stabilization, there are general measures to control raised ICP

that should be done in all patients: head elevation to 30°, maintenance of head and neck in midline position, avoid tight ties around the neck to improve jugular venous drainage, avoid the so called "lethal H" (hypoxia, hypotension, hypercapnia, hyponatremia, hypo and hyperglycemia), and finally early detection and treating of seizures.

Several specific measures have been employed to transient control of cerebral edema and intracranial hypertension. None of them is supported by strong clinical evidence and its role in the treatment of intracranial hypertension is as much as a transient option while surgical treatment is implemented.

Hyperventilation is employed to reduce ICP due to inducing hypocarbia and cerebral vasoconstriction. Because this effect may worse ischemic injury as it was showed in severe head trauma traumatic brain lesions, prophylactic hyperventilation is not recommending and most authors suggest using it for short period of time as rescue maneuver in patients with clinical signs of brain herniation.[51]

Osmotic therapy reduces brain edema by shifting fluids from interstitial and intracellular spaces to intravascular space due to relative osmotic gradient, in areas of brain with intact blood-brain barrier. The main osmotic agents used in clinical setting are mannitol (in a 20% concentration) and hypertonic saline (in concentrations ranging from 3 to 23.4%). A Cochrane review found that the use of mannitol in AIS patients is not supported by evidence from randomized controlled trials.[52] For hypertonic saline the evidence is similar, although a meta-analysis comparing both osmotic agents found greater ICP reductions favoring hypertonic saline despite the small number and size of eligible trials included in the analysis.[53]

Specifically in stroke patients, there is some evidence favor hypertonic saline in reducing raised ICP in patients in which mannitol failed to control it.[54] It is important to note that osmotic therapy should be guided by ICP monitoring and ICP-blinded therapy is not recommended.

Barbiturates are a therapeutic option for treating cerebral edema refractory to other medical measures. There is no evidence of its benefit in the management of increased ICP in stroke patients, added to its association with significant hypotension. For these reasons barbiturate therapy is not recommended to treat cerebral edema in strokes patients.[55]

While these therapies aim to treat edema once it has developed, recent preclinical and phase-2 clinical studies have shown that intravenous glyburide, a Sur-1 receptor inhibitor, blocks edema formation in AIS patients. A randomized clinical trial is ongoing and might contribute to evidence in its clinical benefit.[56]

2) *Surgical treatment of malignant brain edema*: When significant brain swelling occurs in the cerebral hemisphere or cerebellum, surgical decompression should be considered to relieve the mass effect on the middle brain structures and brainstem, and so, avoid major neurological deterioration and death.

There are two scenarios in which surgical treatment has a place in AIS setting: malignant middle cerebral artery (MCA) infarction and cerebellar infarction.

2.1) *Malignant MCA infarction.*

The term refers to a large supratentorial and hemispheric infarct that occurs as a result of a proximal MCA or internal carotid artery occlusion with significant neurological deterioration. There are variable definition criteria for this denomination: NIHSS score > 15–20 points, brain computed tomography ischemic signs involving > 50% of the MCA territory or magnetic resonance diffusion-weighted imaging infarct volume > 145 cc. With best medical treatment, mortality ranges up to 70–80%. The most effective treatment strategy in this context, is decompressive hemicraniectomy (DHC).[15,57,58]

Three randomized clinical trials (DECIMAL, DESTINY and HAMLET) have demonstrated the benefits of early DHC in patients younger than 60 years with malignant cerebral infarct.

A pooled analysis of them showed reduced mortality with DHC compared with medical management (22% versus 71% mortality) and improvement in the percentage of survivors

with good outcomes (mRS score, 0–3: 43% versus 21%).[59,60]

Despite these unequivocal effects on survival and functional outcome, some issues remain uncertain about decompressive craniectomy in ischemic stroke patients:

1. The selection criteria or optimal trigger to perform the DHC. There is an ongoing controversy whether to wait for signs of neurological deterioration, a major midline shift (probably > 5 mm on computed tomography), or whether to operate as soon as the diagnosis of MCA infarction is made. A strategy of "prophylactic" DHC leads to overutilization, whereas policy of waiting for signs of deterioration may aggravate functional outcome. The authors recommend an individualized clinical decision prioritizing early

decompression before signs of herniation occur.[3]

2. Surgical technical aspects have not been clarified at all. The size of the DHC is a very important variable that needs to be addressed, since a size smaller than 12 cm has been linked to poor results and increased cerebral complications, so it must be considered suboptimal. Another aspect is the inclusion of the temporal bone resection at the base, to maximize the decompressive effect of the brainstem. Other surgical decisions, such as the storage of the bone flap have not been prospectively studied.[61]

3. The decision of perform a DHC in patients older than 60 years must take in consideration patients and family wishes, since in this age group DHC can reduce mortality but with a higher likelihood of being severely disabled, as it was showed in the DESTINY II trial.[62,63]

4. Strokectomy or temporal lobectomy could be a potential therapeutic strategy in selected patients who develop clinical failure of DHC. That group of patients characterizes by a persistent and dramatic midline shift after DHC with neurologic deterioration.[64]

2.2) *Cerebellar infarction.*

Cerebellar edema complicates patients with cerebellar infarction in 17 – 54% of cases and is generally related to the posterior inferior cerebellar artery (PICA) territory infarction. A rapid neurological deterioration is typically associated with this situation because the posterior fossa provides a little space for compensation mass effect.

Although, the best surgical approach for malignant cerebellar infarction is a matter of debate, a sub-occipital craniectomy with or without resection of necrotic tissue is recommended after significant cerebellar infarction, in which posterior fossa mass effect produce brainstem distortion, ascending or descending herniation or forth ventricle compression with obstructive acute hydrocephalus.[65,66]

Ventriculostomy should be considered in addition of craniectomy when an obstructive hydrocephalus occurs in this context.

Although the efficacy of surgical treatment of malignant cerebellar infarction has been reported in observational studies, prospective randomized clinical trials will probably never be performed due to depriving affected patients of a life-saving intervention may be considered unethical. In this context, the Statement for Healthcare Professionals from the American Heart Association and American

Stroke Association (AHA/ASA) recommends a suboccipital craniectomy with dural expansion in patients with cerebellar infarctions who deteriorate neurologically despite maximal medical therapy (Class I; Level of Evidence B)[67,68].

10.7 Seizure Prophylaxis

Stroke is one of the main epileptogenic conditions, with an incidence rate of post Stroke epilepsy of 7%[69] and is the first cause of epilepsy in the elderly, accounting for 30 – 50% of all new-onset seizures.[70,71]

Seizure remains as a problematic complication immediately following stroke, because of their unpredictability, unclear effect on prognosis, lack of specific treatment guidelines, increased resources utilization and prolonged length of hospital stay.[72] It has also a negative effect on quality of life through driving restrictions, increased risk of falls and fractures and increased susceptibility to adverse effects from the use of anti-epileptic drugs.[70]

The incidence of post stroke seizure has been reported between 5 – 9% overall.[70,73,74,75,76]

Seizures after stroke can be classified according to their onset in early and late seizures, with clear difference in incidence, pathophysiology and recurrence rate.

Although, International League Against Epilepsy (ILAE, 1981) divided early and late with a cutoff in the first week, most authors recognize as early seizures (ES), those occurring within the first 14 days after acute stroke onset and late onset seizures as occurring after this time window.

More than a half of stroke related seizures occur in the early period, mostly during the first 24 hours, with a reported incidence between 2 – 23%, variably according to different studies. Alvarez et al.[77] in their study limited exclusively to ischemic stroke and acute phase, found an incidence of 1.2% of seizures within the first 7 days after ischemic stroke, all seizures occurred within 72 hours of stroke onset, mostly so within 24 hours, 28.6% at stroke onset and 36.7% within 0.1- 24 hours.

ES after stroke onset are probably the clinical mirror of cortical brain injury, secondary to a cascade of pro-excitatory cellular changes that follow acute ischemic neuronal injury and include glutamate release and accumulation of intracellular $Ca++$ and $Na+$, that promote membrane depolarization and lower threshold. This metabolic dysfunction is self-limited.

On the other hand, late onset seizures are thought to be secondary of gliosis and meningo-cerebral scar, which are permanent structural damage.[75,77,78,79,80,81]

The rate of recurrence or development of epilepsy is higher after late seizures, with an incidence as high as 90%; the reported incidence for ES is relatively low, between 16 – 30%. This difference is probably explained because of the differing pathophysiology.[82]

One of the strongest predictor of seizure occurrence is the cortical involvements.[78] This association has also been demonstrated by Carreras et al[83] in their prospective study based on EEG in acute stroke patients, they found a relation between electrical epileptic activity and cortical lesion.

Other independent risk factor associated with an increase rate of post-stroke ES are stroke severity, size of the infarcts, alcoholism and hemorrhagic transformation.[73,74,78,83,84,85]

Recently, has been linked thrombolysis with rtPA with acute seizures, and was not explained by symptomatic or radiological hemorrhagic transformation, neither by recanalization. This could be the rtPA itself, it is known its neurotoxic effect in vitro and also an epileptogenesis effect in an animal model.[77] Another hypothetical explanations may be recanalization with free-radical production and reperfusion injury that may trigger seizure, with or without hemorrhagic transformation.[86]

Some etiologies, such cardio-embolic (CE) stroke, have been associated for years to ES, but the studies are controversial and this association is not clear right now. Alvarez et al[87] and Stefanidou, M. et al[88] found that the incidence of seizure was similar for CE and large artery atherothrombosis stroke, and in both studies the frequency of seizure for lacunar infarcts was 0%[75,78,81]

The influence of ES after stroke on outcome is controversial. Stroke severity is the strongest determinant of outcome in stroke patients, but it is not know if seizures per se worsen the outcome of ischemic stroke.

Seizures in the acute setting of stroke may worsen outcome by predisposing to aspiration pneumonia, blood pressure fluctuations, increases in ICP or neuronal injury due to increased in metabolic demand. All are secondary injury that might be harmful in already vulnerable tissue, the penumbral area.

Some studies have reported a higher disability/mortality in patients with post-stroke ES [73,75,89,90,91,92] which have not been confirmed by others studies after adjusting for stroke severity.[70,78,84]

The current recommendations, AHA/ASA guidelines 2013 and the European guidelines, are based on the established management of seizures that may complicate any acute brain injury and do not recommend the use of antiepileptic (AE) prophylactic medication[22,93]

There are no recent randomized controlled trials that would answer the question whether antiepileptic drugs (AEDs) have any benefit for primary or secondary prevention of post ischemic stroke seizures.[94]

The use of AEDs can have serious side effects; therefore, their use should be weighed against the risk and morbidity associated with recurrent seizures.

Some studies have found and association between the use of AED-s for secondary seizure prevention and slower motor recovery, worse functional independence and poorer cognitive outcomes[95,96,97,98]

Thrombolysis treatment with rtPA does not prevent the occurrence of ES, according to De Reuck et al, but is probably decreasing the incidence of late seizure. In their group, none of patients treated with rtPA developed recurrence seizure or epilepsy despite the fact that only one patient had been treated with antiepileptic medication.[76]

More studies have to be done to see if any of the reperfusion therapy, rtPA/endovascular thrombectomy, may have any impact in reduce the incidence of post-stroke seizure. According to the differing pathophysiology mechanisms of early and recurrence seizure/epilepsy, we should wait a reduction, mainly, in the incidence of the last one.

Post-stroke seizures are typically controlled by AEDs, in general AED monotherapy is enough to control seizures[75] There is no consensus, though on the appropriate AEDs in post-stroke seizures.

10.8 Temperature Control

Approximately 25 – 40% of patients develops fever (> 37,8 °C) in the first days to 1 week and is commonly associated with neurological deterioration and increased length of stay in the ICU. It is also independently associated with poor outcome, a meta-analysis done by Prasad and Krishnan over 2986 patients, found that patients with AIS and temperature ≥ 37,4 °C within the 24 hours had as twice much mortality than afebrile patients, independent of age and stroke severity.[99]

Fever contributes to disability, through a range of different pathophysiologic mechanisms and its deleterious effect is despite different etiologies, timing of fever and treatments studies.[100] Animal studies have shown that high temperature extend the ischemic area by enhancing free oxygen radical production, exacerbates blood brain barrier breakdown, and worsens cytoskeletal proteolysis.[5]

Knowing the negative impact of hyperthermia in brain injured, its early treatment is the standard of care. First of all, the cause of fever should be sought and specifically treated, being the infection the most common source. Other causes should be kept in mind such as drug fevers and deep venous thrombi. In addition to specific treatment targeting the cause of fever, symptomatic treatment of fever should be immediately done.

There are several strategies for immediate lowering of temperature; these include antipyretics medications, surface cooling and intravascular devices. All these strategies have been use in different studies with the main objective to keep normothermia or even to hypothermia, and see the effect on outcome.

The most common pharmacologic treatment is the use of acetaminophen (mainly in Europe and USA) or non-steroidal anti-inflammatory drug such as ibuprofen.

Recently, the results of the Paracetamol (Acetaminophen) in Stroke (PAIS) trial have been published, which evaluate the empiric administration of acetaminophen to acute stroke patients. They enrolled 1500 (of an intended 2500) patients with baseline temperature 36 – 39 °C. The patients were randomized to acetaminophen 6 g/day versus placebo administered within 12 hours of stroke onset. Even though the treatment with high-dose paracetamol seemed to be safe, there was no significant difference between groups regarding the effect on functional outcome (mRS at 3 months)[101]

Endovascular (venous or arterial) temperature management using feedback devices has been shown effective and safe to keep body temperatures within a narrow range in neurocritical care patients.[102,103] Maintaining prophylactic normothermia with these devices has not shown a significant effect in neurologic outcome yet.

Therapeutic Hypothermia (TH) has been a promising option for patients with ischemic stroke, but the data is not robust enough to consider it as a standard of care in this group of patients. There are no large multicenter clinical trials assessing the benefits on outcome and mortality. The last meta-analysis by Wan et al,[104] reinforced the results showed previously,[105] that TH does not significant improve in stroke severity and mortality.

The current available data about temperature management in AIS is very scarce and the strength of the recommendation is weak. The routine prevention of hyperthermia and the use of induction of hypothermia cannot be recommended as a standard of care. Until future studies elucidate these controversial issues, the recommendation is to treat hyperthermia, avoiding temperature greater than 37.5 °C, and investigate for and treat infectious causes of fever.[1,22,106]

10.9 Glucose Control

Hyperglycemia is an important clinical problem in the acute setting of the stroke. It occurs in more than 40% of patients with or without diabetes previously known.[1,2,5,77]

Acute hyperglycemia (HG) may result secondary to a stress response, preexisting diabetes or from dextrose-containing fluids. Whether HG worsen prognosis or is just a marker of illness severity, is not clear yet. Animal studies have shown that acute hyperglycemia, in a model of focal ischemia; increase neuronal and vascular injury, infarct size, edema, blood brain barrier permeability and the risk of hemorrhagic transformation. It could also contribute to reperfusion injury through impaired autoregulation, exacerbate myogenic dysfunction and impaired effective reperfusion.[107]

Multiple clinical trials have shown the relationship between HG and increased inhospital length of stay (LOS), in-hospital mortality, mortality and morbidity at 90 days, post thrombolysis risk of hemorrhage, and may also attenuate the benefits of intraarterial thrombolysis[6,108,109,110] Two clinical MRI studies measuring the ADC, hyperglycemia and outcome showed a strong association between HG and low ADC, with worse outcome.[111,112] This could be related to a cytotoxic injury exacerbation[111] and the apparition of irreversible ischemic damage within 24 hs in the deep hemispheric white matter, penumbra area, clinically relevant in terms of outcome.[112]

Recently, some published studies, showed higher admission serum glucose and admission hyperglycemia as an independent predictors of adverse outcomes and symptomatic intracerebral hemorrhage in emergent large vessel occlusion (ELVO) patients treated with endovascular therapy/mechanical thrombectomy (MT).[113,114]

Considering all of the above is clear that regular blood glucose monitoring and careful glycemic control is required in all AIS patients, but the specific target serum glucose range to decrease the risk of secondary brain injury is not clear. Neither it is clear the best way to reach the objective range, sliding scale insulin vs. insulin drip.

There are no randomized control trials, which have been shown significant benefit on functional outcome or death, in maintaining tight serum glucose control within a range of 72 – 135 mg/dl with intensive insulin therapy (IIT). Moreover, this strategy significantly increased the number of hypoglycemia episodes.[115,116]

In the INSULINFARCT trial, continuous intravenous insulin infusion provided superior glucose control to subcutaneous insulin, but had no effect on clinical outcome and was paradoxical associated in larger infarct growth.[117]

It seems reasonable to treat HG in a manner that avoids excessive resources, labor and risk. The recommendation for HG until new results of the ongoing trials come out, is to keep blood glucose within 140 – 180 mg/dl in hospitalized patients with AIS[1,4,6,22] and avoid hypoglycemia.

10.10 Venous Thromboembolism Prophylaxis

Venous thromboembolism (VTE), including deep venous thrombosis (DVT) and pulmonary embolism (PE), is a common preventable medical complication in neurocritically ill patients, and account for significant morbidity and mortality. PE accounts for almost 10 – 20% of premature death after stroke in the absence of prophylaxis.

Stroke is associated with an increase risk of DVT. Older age, stroke severity, limb paralysis and dehydration have been documented as risk factors for DVT. An important percentage of the stroke patients have other significant co-morbidities, such as congestive heart failure, atrial fibrillation, and morbid obesity, which increase the risk of this complication.[79,118,119]

The rate of clinically evident DVT and PE in the Stroke population is variably between different studies, with an incidence of 2,5% and 1,2% respectively and this risk persist significant until 4 weeks after stroke.

In a population (n=149916 patients) of AIS patients, enrolled in the Get With The Guidelines-Stroke study, with a rate of DVT prophylaxis of 93%, they found a 2.8% rate of VTE.[118]

The options for thrombo-prophylaxis include early mobilization, systemic antithrombosis/anticoagulation and mechanical devices such as intermittent pneumatic compression (IPC) and graduated stockings.

In the acute setting, the pharmacology-prophylaxis is based on the use of Low Molecular Weight Heparin (LMWH) or un-fractioned heparin (UFH). Both has been demonstrated, by clinical trials and meta-analysis, to significant reduced the risk of DVT, without significantly increase the risk of bleeding, with a slightly better ratio benefit/risk in favor of LMWH[120,121,122]

The Clots in Legs or stocking after Stroke (CLOTS) 3 trial showed that the IPC is an effective and inexpensive method to reduce the risk of DVT (3.6% reduction), and improved survival in immobile stroke patients.[123]

Park et al. in his meta-analysis showed that the use of IPC had a tendency to lowering the DVT risk compared to the control group, but this difference was not significant.

Some of the complications described related with the use of mechanical thromboprophylaxis are: the spread of nosocomial infections, induce mechanical problems of the lower extremity, and dislodge preformed DVT that can result in fatal PE.

All the Acute Stroke Guidelines recommend (▶ Table 10.2) early mobilization as soon as the patient is stable. VTE pharmaco-prophylaxis should be started as soon as feasible in all acute stroke patients. Nyquist et al. recommends dual therapy (pharmacological and mechanical) in patients with restricted immobility, and the use of LMWH over the UFH.

In case of the hemorrhagic transformation of the ischemic stroke, pharmacoprophylaxis should be initiated 24 – 48 hours after the stability of clot according to the CT.

If the patient undergoing hemicraniectomy or endovascular procedure, any form of prophylaxis should be started immediately after the procedure.

Only if the patient has received rtPA the initiation of pharmaco-prophylaxis should be delayed for 24 hours.[4,22,119,124]

In cases of PE from thrombi in the lower extremities and a contraindication for antithrombotic/anticoagulation, placement of a device to filter the inferior vena cava may be considered.

10.11 Gastrointestinal Complications

Gastrointestinal (GI) complications after ischemic stroke are common, with more than 50% of all stroke patients presenting with dysphagia, gastrointestinal bleeding, constipation or fecal incontinence.

All these complications will determine increased hospital length of stay, the development of other complications, and increased mortality.[106,125,126]

Gastrointestinal bleeding: Gastro-duodenal ulcers and GI bleeding are common complications after acute or chronic stages of stroke, and it may interfere with the treatment for ischemic stroke, such as antiplatelet or anticoagulant therapies.

Between 30 – 44% of patients with AIS suffer different types of mucosal injuries, and the reported incidence of GI bleed is between 0.2 – 8%[125,127] The largest study to date with a primary diagnosis of AIS done by Rumalla el al., detected over 3.998.667 patients, an incidence of 1,24% of GI bleeding and 25% of those received blood transfusion.[106]They also found, in a multivariate analysis, a significant association between GI bleeding and increased likelihood of pneumonia, DVT, PE, Urinary Tract Infection, septicemia, acute kidney injury, intubation, tracheostomy, mechanical ventilation, gastrostomy and blood transfusion. Also found an increase of hospital LOS, and in-hospital mortality or severe dependence at discharge. GI bleeding is associated with also increase risk of 6 months and 3 years mortality[127]

The exact pathophysiological mechanism underlying the stress-related mucosa disease is multifactorial. One of the main important factors is splanchnic hypoperfusion due to sympathetic nervous system activation, increased catecholamine released and vasoconstriction. Reductions of gastric mucosal blood flow during ischemic stroke could contribute to ulcerogenesis. Others factor such as systemic inflammation and oxidative stress have also been involved. In animal studies of focal ischemia have been found mucosal endothelial cell necrosis and inflammatory cell infiltration.[128]

Decreased the gastric motility prolongs acid contact time with the gastric mucosa, increasing the risk of ulceration. Side effect of antiplatelet medication is another factor associated to a GI bleeding.[125,129,130]

The American Society of Health System of Pharmacist (ASHP) identified in his guidelines, mechanical ventilation for more than 48 hs and

Table 10.2 DVT prophylaxis	
Early mobilization	As soon as patient stabilized
IPC	As soon as possible
Pharmaco-prophylaxis	As soon as is feasible If Hemorrhagic transformation: once stable clot by CT If hemicraniectomy or endovascular procedure: immediately after If received rtPA: wait 24 hs after the end of the infusion

coagulopathy as the 2 major independent risks factors for GI bleeding in critically ill patients. Other risk factors identified include sepsis, shock, major trauma, spinal cord injury, head injury with GCS less than or equal to 10 or inability to obey command, burn injury (more than 35% of body surface area), corticosteroid therapy (>250 mg of hydrocortisone or equivalent daily).[131]

In studies done in an AIS population the risk factors independently related to increase risk of GI bleeding are previous history of peptic ulcer disease, stroke severity, middle cerebral artery infarcts, increasing age and renal or hepatic dysfunction.[125, 132,133] Rumalla et al. in his results suggested that patients who received thrombolytic therapy for AIS were less likely to suffer from GI bleeding,[133] these has to be confirmed with more studies.

The use of routine gastro-protective drugs as prophylaxis in critically ill patients is still matter of debate. There is a concern above the overuse of stress ulcer prophylaxis (SUP). Farrell et al found that among the group with non-identifiable risk factors for stress related bleeding, 68,1% of them still received SUP. There is a lack of universally accepted standardized guidelines for when initiate or discontinue the stress-ulcer prophylaxis.

The only existing guidelines for SUP were published by the ASHP in 1999, and recommend stress ulcer prophylaxis in the ICU patients when the risk factors described above are present, and should be discontinued when the original risk factor have resolved.[131]

There are no specific recommendations regarding the SUP in the management of AIS guidelines, nor the American neither in the European guidelines.

We recommend SUP in the acute management of ischemic stroke patients who are admitted to an ICU and have any of the risk factor described, ▶ Table 10.3: mechanical ventilation >48 hours,

Table 10.3 Risk factor associated with GI bleeding in AIS and to consider for SUP

Major risk factors	• Mechanical ventilation >48hs • Coagulopathy
Other risk factors	• GCS <11 or inability to follow command • Previous peptic ulcus or GI bleeding • Corticosteroid therapy (>250 mg Hydrocortisone or its equivalent) • Hepatic dysfunction • Renal dysfunction • Severe sepsis

coagulopathy, GCS <11 or inability to follow commands, previous peptic ulcer disease or GI bleeding, corticosteroid therapy (>250 mg of hydrocortisone or equivalent daily), hepatic or renal dysfunction, severe sepsis.

Proton pump inhibitor (PPI) and H2 antagonist have been demonstrated to reduce the risk of GI bleeding, but there is no clear evidence until to date to support the superiority of one over the other.[134,135]

Both drugs have adverse reactions that we should know, such as drug-drug interactions (interacts with cytochrome P450) and altering gastric ph which affect the absorption of various others medications. PPI has been linked with increased risk of Clostridium Difficile nosocomial infection.[88,136] H2 antagonist could cause thrombocytopenia and increased incidence of nosocomial pneumonia.[134,137]

Another important measure to protect against the GI bleeding is *early enteral feeding*. The enteral feeding may prevent GI bleeding by buffering the stomach acid, which may act as a direct source of mucosal energy, induce secretion of cytoprotective prostaglandins mucus and improve mucosal blood flow. A meta-analysis done by Marik et al. suggest that in patients receiving enteral tube feeding, stress ulcer prophylaxis may not be required and indeed, it could increase the risk of complications.[138,139]

Dysphagia is a frequent complication after the stroke, with a prevalence of 45 – 50%, and is significantly related to a stroke severity. It is important an early identification of this dysfunction, because it could be the cause of aspiration pneumonia or post-stroke malnutrition, and it is related to unfavorable outcome, including increase mortality.[125, 140] Stroke secondary to an MCA occlusion or bilateral hemispheric ischemic stroke are associated to a higher incidence of dysphagia. It is suggested, that cerebral ischemia lead to an interruption of the brain-gut axis, and alterations in the neural circuits controlling gastrointestinal.[125]

Most guidelines recommend, a soon as it is possible and depending the patient clinical condition, the use of the water-swallowing test at bedside as a screening for dysphagia. A wet voice swallow is a predictor of high risk for aspiration.[22] This screening can lead to specific recommendation regarding the acute management of stroke, such as nasogastric or naso-duodenal tube placement within the 24 hours after the assessment, to provide early enteral nutrition and facilitates drugs administration. If the patient is intubated and mechanical ventilated it is indicated the use of nasogastric tube and start the enteral nutrition within the 24 hours if not have contraindication.

Others GI complications such as alterations in GI motility have been studied recently in post ischemic stroke. Within this kind of alterations should be considered the dysfunction of the lower esophageal sphincter that could expose the patient to aspirations, vomiting and predict feeding tube failure. Alterations in gastric emptying could also decrease drug absorption. The hypothetical cause of this is the injury to several cortical areas and medullar nuclei involved function and modulation of the autonomic nervous system.[125]

References

[1] McDermott M, Jacobs T, Morgenstern L. Critical care in acute ischemic stroke. Handb Clin Neurol. 2017; 140:153–176

[2] Coplin WM. Critical care management of acute ischemic stroke. Continuum (Minneap Minn). 2012; 18(3):547–559

[3] Torbey MT, Bösel J, Rhoney DH, et al. Evidence-based guidelines for the management of large hemispheric infarction : a statement for health care professionals from the Neurocritical Care Society and the German Society for Neuro-intensive Care and Emergency Medicine. Neurocrit Care. 2015a; 22 (1):146–164

[4] Al-Mufti F, Dancour E, Amuluru K, et al. Neurocritical Care of Emergent Large-Vessel Occlusion. J Intensive Care Med. 2016; 88506661665636. DOI: 10.1177/0885066616656361

[5] Figueroa SA, Zhao W, Aiyagari V. Emergency and critical care management of acute ischaemic stroke. CNS Drugs. 2015; 29(1):17–28

[6] Kirkman MA, Citerio G, Smith M. The intensive care management of acute ischemic stroke: an overview. Intensive Care Med. 2014; 40(5):640–653

[7] Bershad EM, Feen ES, Hernandez OH, Suri MFK, Suarez JI. Impact of a specialized neurointensive care team on outcomes of critically ill acute ischemic stroke patients. Neurocrit Care. 2008; 9(3):287–292

[8] Suarez JI, Zaidat OO, Suri MF, et al. Length of stay and mortality in neurocritically ill patients: impact of a specialized neurocritical care team. Crit Care Med. 2004; 32(11):2311–2317

[9] Rincon F, Mayer SA, Rivolta J, et al. Impact of delayed transfer of critically ill stroke patients from the Emergency Department to the Neuro-ICU. Neurocrit Care. 2010; 13(1):75–81

[10] Burns JD, Green DM, Metivier K, DeFusco C. Intensive care management of acute ischemic stroke. Emerg Med Clin North Am. 2012; 30(3):713–744

[11] Poca MA, Benejam B, Sahuquillo J, et al. Monitoring intracranial pressure in patients with malignant middle cerebral artery infarction: is it useful? J Neurosurg. 2010; 112(3):648–657

[12] Kasner SE. Clinical interpretation and use of stroke scales. Lancet Neurol. 2006; 5(7):603–612

[13] Fountas KN, Kapsalaki EZ, Machinis TG, Boev AN, Robinson JS, Troup EC. Clinical implications of quantitative infrared pupillometry in neurosurgical patients. Neurocrit Care. 2006; 5(1):55–60

[14] Martínez-Ricarte F, Castro A, Poca MA, et al. Infrared pupillometry. Basic principles and their application in the non-invasive monitoring of neurocritical patients. Neurologia. 2013; 28(1):41–51

[15] Jeon S-B, Koh Y, Choi HA, Lee K. Critical care for patients with massive ischemic stroke. J Stroke. 2014; 16(3):146–160

[16] Adler DE, Milhorat TH. The tentorial notch: anatomical variation, morphometric analysis, and classification in 100 human autopsy cases. J Neurosurg. 2002; 96(6):1103–1112

[17] Gökcen E, Caltekin İ, Savrun A, Korkmaz H, Savrun ŞT, Yıldırım G. Alterations in optic nerve sheath diameter according to cerebrovascular disease sub-groups. Am J Emerg Med. 2017; 35(11):1607–1611

[18] Gerriets T, Stolz E, König S, et al. Sonographic monitoring of midline shift in space-occupying stroke: an early outcome predictor. Stroke. 2001; 32(2):442–447

[19] Diedler J, Sykora M, Bast T, et al. Quantitative EEG correlates of low cerebral perfusion in severe stroke. Neurocrit Care. 2009; 11(2):210–216

[20] van Putten MJAM, Tavy DLJ. Continuous quantitative EEG monitoring in hemispheric stroke patients using the brain symmetry index. Stroke. 2004; 35(11):2489–2492

[21] Ali K, Warusevitane A, Lally F, et al. The stroke oxygen pilot study: a randomized controlled trial of the effects of routine oxygen supplementation early after acute stroke–effect on key outcomes at six months. PLoS One. 2013; 8(6):e59274

[22] Jauch EC, Saver JL, Adams HP, Jr, et al. American Heart Association Stroke Council, Council on Cardiovascular Nursing, Council on Peripheral Vascular Disease, Council on Clinical Cardiology. Guidelines for the early management of patients with acute ischemic stroke: a guideline for healthcare professionals from the American Heart Association/American Stroke Association. Stroke. 2013; 44(3):870–947

[23] Rincon F, Kang J, Maltenfort M, et al. Association between hyperoxia and mortality after stroke: a multicenter cohort study. Crit Care Med. 2014; 42(2):387–396

[24] Stringer WA, Hasso AN, Thompson JR, Hinshaw DB, Jordan KG. Hyperventilation-induced cerebral ischemia in patients with acute brain lesions: demonstration by xenon-enhanced CT. AJNR Am J Neuroradiol. 1993; 14(2):475–484

[25] Wang S, Zhang L, Huang K, Lin Z, Qiao W, Pan S. Predictors of extubation failure in neurocritical patients identified by a systematic review and meta-analysis. PLoS One. 2014; 9 (12):e112198

[26] Wendell LC, Raser J, Kasner S, Park S. Predictors of extubation success in patients with middle cerebral artery acute ischemic stroke. Stroke Res Treat. 2011; 2011:248789

[27] Bösel J. Tracheostomy in stroke patients. Curr Treat Options Neurol. 2014; 16(1):274

[28] Villwock JA, Villwock MR, Deshaies EM. Tracheostomy timing affects stroke recovery. J Stroke Cerebrovasc Dis. 2014; 23(5):1069–1072

[29] Schönenberger S, Al-Suwaidan F, Kieser M, Uhlmann L, Bösel J. The SETscore to Predict Tracheostomy Need in Cerebrovascular Neurocritical Care Patients. Neurocrit Care. 2016; 25 (1):94–104

[30] Bösel J, Schiller P, Hook Y, et al. Strokerelated early tracheostomy versus prolonged orotracheal intubation in neurocritical care trial (SETPOINT): A randomized pilot trial. Stroke. 2013; 44(1):21–28

[31] Schönenberger S, Niesen W-D, Fuhrer H, et al. SETPOINT2-Study Group, IGNITE-Study Group. Early tracheostomy in ventilated stroke patients: Study protocol of the international multicentre randomized trial SETPOINT2 (Stroke-related Early Tracheostomy vs. Prolonged Orotracheal

Intubation in Neurocritical care Trial 2). Int J Stroke. 2016; 11(3):368–379

[32] Qureshi AI, Ezzeddine MA, Nasar A, et al. Prevalence of Elevated Blood Pressure in 563,704 Adult Patients Presenting to the Emergency Department with Stroke in the United States. Am J Emerg Med. 2007; 25(1):32–38–. Retrieved from

[33] Leonardi-Bee J, Bath PMW, Phillips SJ, Sandercock PAG, IST Collaborative Group. Blood pressure and clinical outcomes in the International Stroke Trial. Stroke. 2002; 33(5):1315–1320

[34] Liu-DeRyke X, Levy PD, Parker D , Jr, Coplin W, Rhoney DH. A prospective evaluation of labetalol versus nicardipine for blood pressure management in patients with acute stroke. Neurocrit Care. 2013; 19(1):41–47

[35] Delgado-Mederos R, Ribo M, Rovira A, et al. Prognostic significance of blood pressure variability after thrombolysis in acute stroke. Neurology. 2008; 71(8):552–558

[36] Potter JF, Robinson TG, Ford GA, et al. Controlling hypertension and hypotension immediately post-stroke (CHHIPS): a randomised, placebo-controlled, double-blind pilot trial. Lancet Neurol. 2009; 8(1):48–56

[37] Robinson TG, Potter JF, Ford GA, et al. COSSACS Investigators. Effects of antihypertensive treatment after acute stroke in the Continue or Stop Post-Stroke Antihypertensives Collaborative Study (COSSACS): a prospective, randomised, open, blinded-endpoint trial. Lancet Neurol. 2010; 9(8):767–775

[38] Sandset EC, Bath PM, Boysen G, et al. SCAST Study Group. The angiotensin-receptor blocker candesartan for treatment of acute stroke (SCAST): a randomised, placebo-controlled, double-blind trial. Lancet. 2011; 377(9767):741–750

[39] He J, Zhang Y, Xu T, et al. CATIS Investigators. Effects of immediate blood pressure reduction on death and major disability in patients with acute ischemic stroke: the CATIS randomized clinical trial. JAMA. 2014; 311(5):479–489

[40] ENOS Trial Investigators. Efficacy of nitric oxide, with or without continuing antihypertensive treatment, for management of high blood pressure in acute stroke (ENOS): a partial-factorial randomised controlled trial. Lancet. 2015; 385(9968):617–628

[41] Huang Y, Sharma VK, Robinson T, et al. ENCHANTED investigators. Rationale, design, and progress of the ENhanced Control of Hypertension And Thrombolysis stroke study (ENCHANTED) trial: An international multicenter 2×2 quasi-factorial randomized controlled trial of low- vs. standard-dose rt-PA and early intensive vs. International Journal of Stroke: Official Journal of the International Stroke Society. 2015; 10(5):778–788

[42] Mistri AK, Robinson TG, Potter JF. Pressor therapy in acute ischemic stroke: systematic review. Stroke. 2006; 37(6):1565–1571

[43] Xiong L, Liu X, Shang T, et al. Impaired cerebral autoregulation: measurement and application to stroke. J Neurol Neurosurg Psychiatry. 2017; 88(6):520–531

[44] Sheth KN, Sims JR. Neurocritical care and periprocedural blood pressure management in acute stroke. Neurology. 2012; 79(13) Suppl 1:S199–S204

[45] Darki A, Schneck MJ, Agrawal A, Rupani A, Barron JT. Correlation of elevated troponin and echocardiography in acute ischemic stroke. J Stroke Cerebrovasc Dis. 2013; 22(7):959–961

[46] Nguyen H, Zaroff JG. Neurogenic stunned myocardium. Curr Neurol Neurosci Rep. 2009; 9(6):486–491

[47] Prasad A, Lerman A, Rihal CS. Apical ballooning syndrome (Tako-Tsubo or stress cardiomyopathy): a mimic of acute myocardial infarction. Am Heart J. 2008; 155(3):408–417

[48] Micheli S, Agnelli G, Caso V, et al. Acute myocardial infarction and heart failure in acute stroke patients: frequency and influence on clinical outcome. J Neurol. 2012; 259(1):106–110

[49] Tu HTH, Campbell BCV, Churilov L, et al. VISTA collaborators. Frequent early cardiac complications contribute to worse stroke outcome in atrial fibrillation. Cerebrovasc Dis. 2011; 32(5):454–460

[50] Caffes N, Kurland DB, Gerzanich V, Simard JM. Glibenclamide for the treatment of ischemic and hemorrhagic stroke. Int J Mol Sci. 2015; 16(3):4973–4984

[51] Muizelaar JP, Marmarou A, Ward JD, et al. Adverse effects of prolonged hyperventilation in patients with severe head injury: a randomized clinical trial. J Neurosurg. 1991; 75(5):731–739

[52] Bereczki D, Liu M, Fernandes do Prado G, Fekete I. Mannitol for acute stroke. In: Bereczki D, ed. The Cochrane Database of Systematic Reviews. Chichester, UK: John Wiley & Sons, Ltd.; 2001:CD001153

[53] Kamel H, Navi BB, Nakagawa K, Hemphill JC , III, Ko NU. Hypertonic saline versus mannitol for the treatment of elevated intracranial pressure: a meta-analysis of randomized clinical trials. Crit Care Med. 2011; 39(3):554–559

[54] Schwarz S, Georgiadis D, Aschoff A, Schwab S. Effects of hypertonic (10%) saline in patients with raised intracranial pressure after stroke. Stroke. 2002; 33(1):136–140

[55] Schwab S, Spranger M, Schwarz S, Hacke W. Barbiturate coma in severe hemispheric stroke: useful or obsolete? Neurology. 1997; 48(6):1608–1613

[56] Sheth KN, Elm JJ, Molyneaux BJ, et al. Safety and efficacy of intravenous glyburide on brain swelling after large hemispheric infarction (GAMES-RP): a randomised, double-blind, placebo-controlled phase 2 trial. Lancet Neurol. 2016; 15(11):1160–1169

[57] Godoy D, Piñero G, Cruz-Flores S, Alcalá Cerra G, Rabinstein A. Malignant hemispheric infarction of the middle cerebral artery. Diagnostic considerations and treatment options. Neurologia. 2016; 31(5):332–343

[58] Hacke W, Schwab S, Horn M, Spranger M, De Georgia M, von Kummer R. 'Malignant' middle cerebral artery territory infarction: clinical course and prognostic signs. Arch Neurol. 1996; 53(4):309–315

[59] Jüttler E, Schellinger PD, Aschoff A, Zweckberger K, Unterberg A, Hacke W. Clinical review: Therapy for refractory intracranial hypertension in ischaemic stroke. Crit Care. 2007; 11(5):231

[60] Vahedi K, Hofmeijer J, Juettler E, et al. DECIMAL, DESTINY, and HAMLET investigators. Early decompressive surgery in malignant infarction of the middle cerebral artery: a pooled analysis of three randomised controlled trials. Lancet Neurol. 2007; 6(3):215–222

[61] Park J, Kim E, Kim G-J, Hur Y-K, Guthikonda M. External decompressive craniectomy including resection of temporal muscle and fascia in malignant hemispheric infarction. J Neurosurg. 2009; 110(1):101–105

[62] Jüttler E, Unterberg A, Woitzik J, et al. DESTINY II Investigators. Hemicraniectomy in older patients with extensive middle-cerebral-artery stroke. N Engl J Med. 2014; 370(12):1091–1100

[63] Weil AG, Rahme R, Moumdjian R, Bouthillier A, Bojanowski MW. Quality of life following hemicraniectomy for malignant MCA territory infarction. Can J Neurol Sci. 2011; 38(3):434–438

[64] Merenda A, Perez-Barcena J, Frontera G, Benveniste RJ. Predictors of clinical failure of decompressive hemicraniectomy for malignant hemispheric infarction. J Neurol Sci. 2015; 355(1–2):54–58

[65] Jauss M, Krieger D, Hornig C, Schramm J, Busse O. Surgical and medical management of patients with massive cerebellar infarctions: results of the German-Austrian Cerebellar Infarction Study. J Neurol. 1999; 246(4):257–264

[66] Tsitsopoulos PP, Tobieson L, Enblad P, Marklund N. Surgical treatment of patients with unilateral cerebellar infarcts: clinical outcome and prognostic factors. Acta Neurochir (Wien). 2011; 153(10):2075–2083

[67] Jüttler E, Schwab S, Schmiedek P, et al. DESTINY Study Group. Decompressive surgery for the treatment of malignant infarction of the middle cerebral artery (DESTINY): A randomized, controlled trial. Stroke. 2007; 38(9):2518–2525

[68] Wijdicks EFM, Sheth KN, Carter BS, et al. American Heart Association Stroke Council. Recommendations for the management of cerebral and cerebellar infarction with swelling: a statement for healthcare professionals from the American Heart Association/American Stroke Association. Stroke. 2014; 45(4):1222–1238

[69] Zhou B, Huang Y, Wang J, et al. The aetiology of convulsive status epilepticus: a study of 258 cases in Western China. Seizure. 2014; 23(9):717–721

[70] Reith J, Jørgensen HS, Nakayama H, Raaschou HO, Olsen TS. Seizures in acute stroke: predictors and prognostic significance. The Copenhagen Stroke Study. Stroke. 1997; 28(8):1585–1589

[71] Tanaka T, Ihara M. Post-stroke epilepsy. Neurochem Int. 2016; 5–7. DOI: 10.1016/j.neuint.2017.02.002

[72] Huang C-W, Saposnik G, Fang J, Steven DA, Burneo JG. Influence of seizures on stroke outcomes: a large multicenter study. Neurology. 2014; 82(9):768–776

[73] Bladin CF, Alexandrov AV, Bellavance A, et al. Seizures after stroke: a prospective multicenter study. Arch Neurol. 2000; 57(11):1617–1622

[74] Bladin CF, Bornstein N. Post-stroke seizures. Handb Clin Neurol. 2009; 93:613–621

[75] Bryndziar T, Sedova P, Kramer NM, et al. Seizures Following Ischemic Stroke: Frequency of Occurrence and Impact on Outcome in a Long-Term Population-Based Study. J Stroke Cerebrovasc Dis. 2016; 25(1):150–156

[76] De Reuck J, Van Maele G. Acute ischemic stroke treatment and the occurrence of seizures. Clin Neurol Neurosurg. 2010; 112(4):328–331

[77] Alvarez V. Acute seizures in the acute ischemic stroke setting: a step forward in their description. Neurology. 2014; 82(9):740–741

[78] Alberti A, Paciaroni M, Caso V, Venti M, Palmerini F, Agnelli G. Early seizures in patients with acute stroke: frequency, predictive factors, and effect on clinical outcome. Vasc Health Risk Manag. 2008; 4(3):715–720

[79] Bustamante A, García-Berrocoso T, Rodriguez N, et al. Ischemic stroke outcome: A review of the influence of post-stroke complications within the different scenarios of stroke care. Eur J Intern Med. 2016; 29:9–21

[80] Silverman IE, Restrepo L, Mathews GC. Poststroke seizures. Arch Neurol. 2002; 59(2):195–201

[81] Stefanidou M, Das RR, Beiser AS, et al. Incidence of seizures following initial ischemic stroke in a community-based cohort: The Framingham Heart Study. Seizure. 2017; 47:105–110

[82] De Reuck J, De Groote L, Van Maele G, Katsarou N, Back T, Vescovi M. Single seizure and epilepsy in patients with a cerebral territorial infarct. J Neurol Sci. 2008; 271(1–2):127–130

[83] Carrera E, Michel P, Despland PA, et al. Continuous assessment of electrical epileptic activity in acute stroke. Neurology. 2006; 67(1):99–104

[84] Labovitz DL, Hauser WA, Sacco RL. Prevalence and predictors of early seizure and status epilepticus after first stroke. Neurology. 2001; 57(2):200–206

[85] Zhang C, Wang X, Wang Y, et al. Risk factors for post-stroke seizures: a systematic review and meta-analysis. Epilepsy Res. 2014; 108(10):1806–1816

[86] Rodan LH, Aviv RI, Sahlas DJ, Murray BJ, Gladstone JP, Gladstone DJ. Seizures during stroke thrombolysis heralding dramatic neurologic recovery. Neurology. 2006; 67(11):2048–2049

[87] Alvarez V, Rossetti AO, Papavasileiou V, Michel P. Acute seizures in acute ischemic stroke: does thrombolysis have a role to play? J Neurol. 2013; 260(1):55–61

[88] Aseeri M, Schroeder T, Kramer J, Zackula R. Gastric acid suppression by proton pump inhibitors as a risk factor for clostridium difficile-associated diarrhea in hospitalized patients. Am J Gastroenterol. 2008; 103(9):2308–2313

[89] Arboix A, Comes E, García-Eroles L, Massons JB, Oliveres M, Balcells M. Prognostic value of very early seizures for in-hospital mortality in atherothrombotic infarction. Eur Neurol. 2003; 50(2):78–84

[90] Arboix A, García-Eroles L, Massons JB, Oliveres M, Comes E. Predictive factors of early seizures after acute cerebrovascular disease. Stroke. 1997; 28(8):1590–1594

[91] Jung S, Schindler K, Findling O, et al. Adverse effect of early epileptic seizures in patients receiving endovascular therapy for acute stroke. Stroke. 2012; 43(6):1584–1590

[92] Lamy C, Domigo V, Semah F, et al. Patent Foramen Ovale and Atrial Septal Aneurysm Study Group. Early and late seizures after cryptogenic ischemic stroke in young adults. Neurology. 2003; 60(3):400–404

[93] Alonso de Leciñana M., Egido J. A., Casado I.. Guía para el tratamiento del infarto cerebral agudo. Neurologia. 2014; 29 (2):102–122

[94] Sykes L, Wood E, Kwan J, Kwan J. Antiepileptic drugs for the primary and secondary prevention of seizures after stroke. Cochrane Database Syst Rev. 2014(1):CD005398

[95] Goldstein LB, The Sygen In Acute Stroke Study Investigators. Common drugs may influence motor recovery after stroke. Neurology. 1995; 45(5):865–871

[96] Kulhari A, Strbian D, Sundararajan S. Early onset seizures in stroke. Stroke. 2014; 45(12):e249–e251

[97] Naidech AM, Kreiter KT, Janjua N, et al. Phenytoin exposure is associated with functional and cognitive disability after subarachnoid hemorrhage. Stroke. 2005; 36(3):583–587

[98] Ryvlin P, Montavont A, Nighoghossian N. Optimizing therapy of seizures in stroke patients. Neurology. 2006; 67(12) Suppl 4:S3–S9

[99] Prasad K, Krishnan PR. Fever is associated with doubling of odds of short-term mortality in ischemic stroke: an updated meta-analysis. Acta Neurol Scand. 2010; 122(6):404–408

[100] Marehbian J, Greer DM. Normothermia and Stroke. Curr Treat Options Neurol. 2017; 19(1):4

[101] de Ridder IR, den Hertog HM, van Gemert HMA, et al. Trial Organization. PAIS 2 (Paracetamol [Acetaminophen] in Stroke 2): Results of a Randomized, Double-Blind Placebo-Controlled Clinical Trial. Stroke. 2017; 48(4):977–982

[102] Broessner G, Beer R, Lackner P, et al. Prophylactic, endovascularly based, long-term normothermia in ICU patients with severe cerebrovascular disease: bicenter prospective, randomized trial. Stroke. 2009; 40(12):e657–e665

[103] Fischer M, Lackner P, Beer R, et al. Cooling Activity is Associated with Neurological Outcome in Patients with Severe

Cerebrovascular Disease Undergoing Endovascular Temperature Control. Neurocrit Care. 2015; 23(2):205–209

[104] Wan Y-H, Nie C, Wang H-L, Huang C-Y. Therapeutic hypothermia (different depths, durations, and rewarming speeds) for acute ischemic stroke: a meta-analysis. J Stroke Cerebrovasc Dis. 2014; 23(10):2736–2747

[105] Lakhan SE, Pamplona F. Application of mild therapeutic hypothermia on stroke: a systematic review and meta-analysis. Stroke Res Treat. 2012; 2012:295906

[106] Ntaios G, Papavasileiou V, Bargiota A, Makaritsis K, Michel P. Intravenous insulin treatment in acute stroke: a systematic review and meta-analysis of randomized controlled trials. Int J Stroke. 2014; 9(4):489–493

[107] Hafez S, Coucha M, Bruno A, Fagan SC, Ergul A. Hyperglycemia, acute ischemic stroke, and thrombolytic therapy. Transl Stroke Res. 2014; 5(4):442–453

[108] Bruno A, Levine SR, Frankel MR, et al. NINDS rt-PA Stroke Study Group. Admission glucose level and clinical outcomes in the NINDS rt-PA Stroke Trial. Neurology. 2002; 59(5):669–674

[109] Fuentes B, Castillo J, San José B, et al. Stroke Project of the Cerebrovascular Diseases Study Group, Spanish Society of Neurology. The prognostic value of capillary glucose levels in acute stroke: the GLycemia in Acute Stroke (GLIAS) study. Stroke. 2009; 40(2):562–568

[110] Gofir A, Mulyono B, Sutarni S. Hyperglycemia as a prognosis predictor of length of stay and functional outcomes in patients with acute ischemic stroke. Int J Neurosci. 2017; 127(10):923–929

[111] Bevers MB, Vaishnav NH, Pham L, Battey TW, Kimberly WT. Hyperglycemia is associated with more severe cytotoxic injury after stroke. J Cereb Blood Flow Metab. 2017; 37(7):2577–2583

[112] Rosso C, Pires C, Corvol J-C, et al. Hyperglycaemia, insulin therapy and critical penumbral regions for prognosis in acute stroke: further insights from the INSULINFARCT trial. PLoS One. 2015; 10(3):e0120230

[113] Goyal N, Tsivgoulis G, Pandhi A, et al. Admission hyperglycemia and outcomes in large vessel occlusion strokes treated with mechanical thrombectomy. J Neurointerv Surg. 2017; •••:2017–012993

[114] Sugiura Y, Yamagami H, Sakai N, Yoshimura S, Committee of Recovery by Endovascular Salvage for Cerebral Ultra-acute Embolism (RESCUE)-Japan Study Group. Predictors of Symptomatic Intracranial Hemorrhage after Endovascular Therapy in Acute Ischemic Stroke with Large Vessel Occlusion. J Stroke Cerebrovasc Dis. 2017; 26(4):766–771

[115] Bellolio MF, Gilmore RM, Ganti L. Insulin for glycaemic control in acute ischaemic stroke. Cochrane Database Syst Rev. 2014(1):CD005346

[116] Ntaios G, Dziedzic T, Michel P, et al. European Stroke Organisation. European Stroke Organisation (ESO) guidelines for the management of temperature in patients with acute ischemic stroke. Int J Stroke. 2015; 10(6):941–949

[117] Rosso C, Corvol J-C, Pires C, et al. Intensive versus subcutaneous insulin in patients with hyperacute stroke: results from the randomized INSULINFARCT trial. Stroke. 2012; 43(9):2343–2349

[118] Douds GL, Hellkamp AS, Olson DM, et al. Venous thromboembolism in the Get With The Guidelines-Stroke acute ischemic stroke population: incidence and patterns of prophylaxis. J Stroke Cerebrovasc Dis. 2014; 23(1):123–129

[119] Nyquist P, Jichici D, Bautista C, et al. Prophylaxis of Venous Thrombosis in Neurocritical Care Patients: An Executive Summary of Evidence-Based Guidelines: A Statement for Healthcare Professionals From the Neurocritical Care Society and Society of Critical Care Medicine. Crit Care Med. 2017; 45(3):476–479

[120] Kamphuisen PW, Agnelli G. What is the optimal pharmacological prophylaxis for the prevention of deep-vein thrombosis and pulmonary embolism in patients with acute ischemic stroke? Thromb Res. 2007; 119(3):265–274

[121] Park J, Lee JM, Lee JS, Cho Y-J. Pharmacological and Mechanical Thromboprophylaxis in Critically Ill Patients: a Network Meta-Analysis of 12 Trials. J Korean Med Sci. 2016; 31(11):1828–1837

[122] Sherman DG, Albers GW, Bladin C, et al. PREVAIL Investigators. The efficacy and safety of enoxaparin versus unfractionated heparin for the prevention of venous thromboembolism after acute ischaemic stroke (PREVAIL Study): an open-label randomised comparison. Lancet. 2007; 369(9570):1347–1355

[123] Dennis M, Sandercock P, Graham C, Forbes J, Smith J, CLOTS (Clots in Legs Or sTockings after Stroke) Trials Collaboration. The Clots in Legs Or sTockings after Stroke (CLOTS) 3 trial: a randomised controlled trial to determine whether or not intermittent pneumatic compression reduces the risk of post-stroke deep vein thrombosis and to estimate its cost-effectiveness. Health Technol Assess. 2015; 19(76):1–90

[124] Powers WJ, Derdeyn CP, Biller J, et al. American Heart Association Stroke Council. 2015 American Heart Association/American stroke association focused update of the 2013 guidelines for the early management of patients with acute ischemic stroke regarding endovascular treatment: A guideline for healthcare professionals from the American. Stroke. 2015; 46(10):3020–3035

[125] Camara-Lemarroy CR, Ibarra-Yruegas BE, Gongora-Rivera F. Gastrointestinal complications after ischemic stroke. J Neurol Sci. 2014; 346(1–2):20–25

[126] Rumalla K, Mittal MK. Gastrointestinal Bleeding in Acute Ischemic Stroke: A Population-Based Analysis of Hospitalizations in the United States. J Stroke Cerebrovasc Dis. 2016; 25(7):1728–1735

[127] Chou Y-F, Weng W-C, Huang W-Y. Association between gastrointestinal bleeding and 3-year mortality in patients with acute, first-ever ischemic stroke. J Clin Neurosci. 2017; 44:289–293

[128] Hung C-R. Role of gastric oxidative stress and nitric oxide in formation of hemorrhagic erosion in rats with ischemic brain. World J Gastroenterol. 2006; 12(4):574–581. Retrieved from www.wjgnet.com

[129] Feng G, Xu X, Wang Q, Liu Z, Li Z, Liu G. The protective effects of calcitonin gene-related peptide on gastric mucosa injury after cerebral ischemia reperfusion in rats. Regul Pept. 2010; 160(1–3):121–128

[130] Tseng CK, Tsai CH, Tseng CH, Tseng YC, Lee FY, Huang WS. An outbreak of foodborne botulism in Taiwan. Int J Hyg Environ Health. 2009; 212(1):82–86

[131] ASHP Therapeutic Guidelines on Stress Ulcer Prophylaxis. ASHP Therapeutic Guidelines on Stress Ulcer Prophylaxis. ASHP Commission on Therapeutics and approved by the ASHP Board of Directors on November 14, 1998. Am J Health Syst Pharm. 1999; 56(4):347–379

[132] Hamidon BB, Raymond AA. The risk factors of gastrointestinal bleeding in acute ischaemic stroke. Med J Malaysia. 2006; 61(3):288–291

[133] Rumalla K, Kumar AS, Mittal MK. Gastrointestinal Bowel Obstruction in Acute Ischemic Stroke: Incidence, Risk Factors, and Outcomes in a U.S. Nationwide Analysis of 3,998,667 Hospitalizations. J Stroke Cerebrovasc Dis. 2017; 26(10):2093–2101

[134] Anderson ME. Stress Ulcer Prophylaxis in Hospitalized Patients. Hosp Med Clin. 2013; 2:e32–e44

[135] Barletta JF, Bruno JJ, Buckley MS, Cook DJ. Stress Ulcer Prophylaxis. Crit Care Med. 2016; 44(7):1395–1405

[136] Loo VG, Bourgault A-M, Poirier L, et al. Host and pathogen factors for Clostridium difficile infection and colonization. N Engl J Med. 2011; 365(18):1693–1703. Retrieved from

[137] Farrell CP, Mercogliano G, Kuntz CL. Overuse of stress ulcer prophylaxis in the critical care setting and beyond. J Crit Care. 2010; 25(2):214–220

[138] Avendaño-Reyes JM, Jaramillo-Ramírez H. [Prophylaxis for stress ulcer bleeding in the intensive care unit]. Rev Gastroenterol Mex. 2014; 79(1):50–55

[139] Marik PE, Vasu T, Hirani A, Pachinburavan M. Stress ulcer prophylaxis in the new millennium: a systematic review and meta-analysis. Crit Care Med. 2010; 38(11):2222–2228

[140] Crary MA, Carnaby-Mann GD, Miller L, Antonios N, Silliman S. Dysphagia and nutritional status at the time of hospital admission for ischemic stroke. J Stroke Cerebrovasc Dis. 2006; 15(4):164–171

11 Stroke in Pediatric Population

Roberto Crosa

Abstract
The incidence of pediatric stroke is low, but this underdiagnosed disease is included among the 10 most frequent causes of death in children. The clinical picture is non-specific: seizures in the newborn, focal symptoms in older children and teenagers. Stroke of venous origin may associate intracranial hypertension. Ischemic stroke is more frequent. Etiology varies widely: infection, heart disease, prothrombotic conditions of diverse origin, arterial trauma and congenital metabolic defects. A modification of the NIHSS score, the pedNIHss score, can be used in children 2 to 18 years of age on their arrival at the hospital. Diagnosis is usually delayed, which could be compensated by prompt MRI. CT being more readily available, it is generally done first although it is less precise. MR has more scope, it can differentiate stroke from other neurological diseases, but it requires sedation. For arterial pathology, DSA is the method of choice for arterial pathology, whether cervical or intracranial. Stabilization in the acute stage may include hydration and anticonvulsants. Fibrinolytics are ineffective. LMWH is often used, on empirical grounds. Corticosteroids might be of benefit in ischemic strokes of infectious origin. If cranial sutures are closed, intracranial hypertension might occur and call for early decompressive craniectomy, especially in cases of malignant ischemic infarction in the MCA or ICA territories.

Keywords: pediatric stroke, intracranial hypertension, ischemic stroke, DSA as a method of choice, MRI as a method of choice, malignant ischemic infarction in MCA territory

11.1 Introduction and Epidemiology

It is a real challenge to write a chapter on pediatric stroke, given that available information, experience, and scientific evidence are quite limited. As opposed to the approach to stroke in the adult population, the approach to stroke in childhood often lacks a clear scientific outline, being based on small case series and reports of isolated cases. There have, however, been reports of ischemic stroke cases in children as far back as the eighteenth century.

Approaching this entity as a single condition is always a problem. It should be envisaged differently for each stage, because causes, symptoms and prognoses are different at each stage of childhood. As opposed to general opinion, pediatric stroke is among the top 10 causes of death in children in the United States.[1] It occurs much oftener than is generally thought, incidence being between 2, 3 to 13 in 100,000 children. From a historic point of view, this incidence is on the rise, perhaps due to more awareness of the problem (and subsequently, more specialists suspecting this diagnosis) and also to the fact that patients at risk for stroke live longer now.[2,3] Another important contributing factor is progress in imaging techniques that diagnose stroke cases. Some of these techniques are increasingly common, like MRI.

Unfortunately it looks like pediatric stroke is still underestimated in spite of its frequency. In most of the cases that have come our way we have observed a low level of suspicion, with the subsequent delay in diagnosis that goes beyond 24 hours, as will be discussed later.

Stroke is so frequent that it even competes with tumors of the central nervous system in pediatrics for the first places in incidence lists. Although in most case reports on this subject patients are older than 28 days, it is 17 times more frequent in newborn period; in this population, a stroke is especially likely to occur.

As opposed to the situation in the adult population, AIS incidence is slightly higher than the incidence of acute hemorrhagic stroke. There is a clear male predominance, approximately 60%. There are clear epidemiological ethnic differences that have not been well defined so far.[4]

On facing a pediatric patient with AIS, marked differences with adult cases appear. That is why we have decided to write a separate chapter about this group. Not only is AIS more frequent than hemorrhagic stroke, there is also a noticeable arterial-venous ratio of 3/1 as a cause for ischemic stroke in children. The ratio in newborns is 2/1.[5] Venous pathology, then, plays a great role in this often-forgotten disease of children. Nonspecific symptoms associated with stroke must ALWAYS awaken suspicion of this disease in a child with nonspecific neurological symptomatology.

11.2 Clinical Symptoms

The clinical manifestations of stroke in childhood are clearly linked to the corresponding stage in the child's life. It becomes difficult, therefore, to organize this complex subject.

Cases of intrauterine stroke have long been known and reported[6] but always as isolated cases with no evident symptoms, which were diagnosed on account of clinical manifestations days or weeks after birth or as autopsy findings in children who died soon after birth.

The symptoms may appear suddenly or gradually, they may associate neurological impairment or not, they may include seizures, etc., according not only to the cause but to the age of the patient.

In the newborn period, ischemic stroke tends to present with seizure and rarely, if ever, with any noticeable focal neurological deficit. The onset is usually insidious, which is not the case with older children. Focal neurological deficits become more apparent from a few monthsto a year later.

According to some reports, evident signs of neurological deficit that are related to perinatal or neonatal brain ischemia may be delayed. In 18 out of 22 cases, lack of use of one hand is related to probable perinatal ischemia, while in 12 out of 22 cases, permanent alterations of language, cognition or behavior develop during a long-term follow-up.[7]

In children older than one year, early and unusual dominance of one hand may indicate a previous stroke. The disease may still appear associated with seizures, fever or coma. This symptomatology becomes less frequent as children get older. Adolescents present more regularly with acute-onset hemiparesia, with or without seizures, a clinical picture that often regresses. Fever, seizures, and headaches are less frequent.[8]

Stage of childhood is not the only determining cause; other factors and the affected territory also play a role in the presentation of symptoms. In the case of ischemic arterial strokes, the affectation of proximal arteries in the anterior sector is better tolerated than in adults, perhaps because vascular anastomotic circuits, intracranial and extracranial, are notoriously more present. The incidence of such anterior strokes is supposed to reach 71% of cases in children. It should be underlined that in 8% of cases both anterior territories are associated,[9] which is a remarkable phenomenon.

Venous strokes are apt to have a more insidious, progressive and unspecific onset, and they are associated to vague symptomatology. Intracranial hypertension may be associated. Focal symptoms are not always present, and they depend on the affected territory, which is nearly impossible to diagnose by clinical means only. Some symptomatologic associations linked to brain venous thromboses have been described, but the latter do not always result in symptoms, because of the particular complexity of brain anatomy and venous hemodynamics in children.

Transitory ischemic attacks do not present with lipohyalinosis as in adults; if they occur at all, they are associated with hemiplegic migraine or other manifestations of brain insufficiency due to moyamoya disease (which increases brain metabolic requirements) or to arteriovenous fistulae originating a local circulatory steal phenomenon.

11.3 Etiology

The causes of ischemic stroke in childhood are invariably manifold and not well-known. In most cases (80%), however, a specific cause for stroke can be found if the case is adequately studied.

The study of risk factors is most important in these cases in order to understand and supervise the great amount of lab tests and imaging that will be suggested.

According to the Canadian Pediatric Ischemic Stroke Registry (2017), nearly half the cases of stroke develop in previously healthy children, but in newborns, strokes are part of an acute systemic disease (infectious or not), arise in prothrombotic conditions, or are a consequence of maternal disorders. Outside the newborn period, other more specific pediatric factors come into play, like arteriopathy (50%), congenital or acquired heart disease (24%), and prothrombotic or hematological disorder (20–50%). There may be a previous trauma, especially in cases of arterial dissection and also in some venous cerebral thromboses.[10,11]

Venous conditions usually are associated with infections, dehydration, head trauma or congenital prothrombotic states. In sum, 50% of the cases associate with a risk factor, 75% with more than one and in 25% no risk factors are to be found.[4]

In order to diagnose correctly, the fundamental steps are: a painstaking case history, a careful physical examination (it must be borne in mind, however, that this is a neurological emergency), then specific imaging, adequate cardiological assessment and a complete study of coagulation. In children it is especially important to differentiate conditions of venous etiology from those of arterial etiology, as well as thrombotic disorders

Table 11.1 Etiology of ischemic stroke in childhood

Arterial and Venous Occlusion	Venous Occlusion	No Occlusion
Hematological diseases (congenital thrombophilia, drepanocytosis, antiphospholipidic syndrome)	Septic thrombophlebitis	Decrease of cardiac output
Arterial dissection	Aseptic thrombophlebitis	Circulatory steal phenomena (AVM)
Infectious vasculitis (bacterial, viral and fungal)		
Noninfectious vasculitis (Lupus, Takayasu, Polyarteritis nodosa, juvenile rheumatoid arthritis, Kawasaki disease)		
Primitive vasculopathies (moyamoya, fibromuscular dysplasia)		
Drugs (cocaine, anphetamines)		
Metabolic diseases (hyperhomocysteinemia, ornithine transcarbamylase deficiency, methylmalonic acidemia, MELAS)		
Ssytemic vascular diseases		
Embolisms: cardiopathies		

from embolic disorders, as shown in table
► Table 11.1

Congenital cyanotic cardiopathies are a common cause of stroke in children, on account of their compensating polycytemia's determining both local thrombosis (arterial or venous) and arterial embolism. Acquired cardiopathies are also a relatively frequent cause of embolism in brain arteries. This applies to both valvular disease like rheumatic disease, mitral prolapse, auricular myxoma, valvular prostheses and myocardial disease, like myocardiopathies and arrhythmias.

Traumatic intracranial arterial conditions, classically considered infrequent, deserve a whole new chapter. They are thought to be one of the leading causes of stroke in childhood, particularly in older children.[12] Basically, dissections can be divided into intracranial or extracranial, and may in turn be either subintimal or subadventitial. Through a lesion of the intima of a cerebral artery blood enters between the intima and the media layer. As a consequence, the arterial lumen becomes narrower, and blood flow is reduced. Distal embolism may arise from that lesion. Once blood forces its way through the whole media layer, the dissection becomes adventitial, and there is risk of both ischemic and hemorrhagic stroke; those are extremely severe cases with high morbimortality.

Arterial dissections have always been linked to previous trauma, but we often see in practice that this event does not appear clearly in the case history and therefore stroke goes unsuspected and undiagnosed, with the subsequent loss of time while investigating wrong etiologies.

It must be remembered, too, that a third of strokes in childhood occur in the context of infection, viral or bacterial. Arterial vasculitis can originate stroke in children. Numerous agents like nonspecific bacteria, tuberculous bacilli, Mycoplasma, Chlamydia, herpesvirus, HIV and fungus can cause arterial vasculitis when they invade the central nervous system (CNS). Meningitis often associates venous thrombosis of cortical and deep communicant veins, while HNT infections tend to affect the transverse sinuses, the sphenoparietal sinuses of Brechet and the cavernous sinus that run through the region.

Nevertheless vasculitis is not a particularly frequent cause of ischemic stroke in children, as opposed to what is generally assumed.

Hematological diseases may cause brain infarcts, either arterial or venous. Both acquired hematological disorders (like disseminated erythematosus lupus and iatrogenic diseases) and congenital hematological conditions (such as hereditary deficiency of coagulation inhibitors, such as proteins C or S or antithrombin III, increase of clotting proteins or mutations of the prothrombin gene) increase the possibility of ischemic stroke on account of hypercoagulability or a prethrombotic state. They constitute a clear risk for stroke in childhood.

Nearly 4% of the population has a mutation of the prothrombin gene (20210) and 2 to 15% of the white population evidences a resistance to natural clotting of activated protein C, which is associated with a mutation of the factor V Leiden. Both circumstances dramatically increase the occurrence of thrombosis in that population. In these pro-thrombotic cases, both veins and arteries of the brain are diseased.[13]

Hyperhomocysteinemia is a well-known risk factor for stroke in children. The mechanism involves a C677T mutation that produces a 5–10 methytetrahydrofolate reductase (MTHFR) variant, which in turn decreases the amount of available 1.5-methyltetrahydrofolate for the conversion of homocystein into methionine.

An increase in lipoprotein (a) can result in pro-thrombotic states because it competes with plas-minogen; it inhibits fibrinolysis and increases the risk of thrombosis.

Deficiency of proteins C and S may be acquired, for example by sepsis and viral infections like varicella.

Other prothrombotic abnormalities less fre-quently associated with ischemic stroke are thrombocytosis, dysfibrinogenemia and increase of factor VIII.[13]

Such prothrombotic alterations may coincide with other events favoring thrombosis (arterial or venous manipulation, infections, sideropenic anemia), thus clearly boosting the risk for ischemic stroke.

The Registry of the Canadian Stroke Network evidences a clear increase of risk for patients with a mutation of factor V Leiden, high levels of lipo-protein (a) or a deficiency of protein C and anti-phospholipid antibodies.[13] An association of these factors obviously heightens the risk of an ischemic stroke occurring in childhood.

The association of other pathological entities can also increase the risk for stroke in children. That is the case with falciform anemia, noninfectious immunologic vasculitis as part of a connective tis-sue disease (such as systemic lupus erythematosus, polyarteritis nodosa, Henoch-Schönlein purpura, Takayasu arteritis), fibromuscular dysplasia, meta-bolic diseases (such as ornithine transcarbamylase deficiency, methylmalonic aciduria and MELAS) and moyamoya disease. Detailed analysis of these dis-eases falls beyond the scope of this chapter.

11.4 Stroke Severity Score

The National Institutes of Health Stroke Scale (NIHSS) is a quantitative scale of great predictive value for the assessment of stroke severity and long-term outcomes. Expert pediatricians and adult stroke specialists arrived at a consensus pediatric score called PedNHISS, which is a modi-fied version of of the NIHSS scale, adjusted accord-ing to the cognitive and neurological development of pediatric patients. This pediatric stroke scale, which can be appropriately used in children aged 2 to 8 years, is the most recommended clinical scale for patient assessment on arrival at the hos-pital, in order to evaluate the result of treatments in each case.[14]

11.5 Diagnostic Delay in Pediatric Stroke

Diagnostic delay for stroke in children is more than three times the delay in adults. A Canadian cohort study demonstrated in 2009 that the average diag-nostic delay was between 22.7 hours and 11.6 hours for hospitalized patients and 29 hours for outpatients. Against expectations, delay at the patient's house amounted only to 1.7 hours.[15] This fact underlines that the main problem related to this especially sensitive topic relates to hospital arrival: on account of several circumstances diag-nosis is not reached in time when children are concerned. In 2002, a retrospective study on 29 children affected by stroke showed a diagnostic delay of 35 hours. A later review found that out of 50 pediatric stroke cases, 32 patients were not seen by a neurologist in the first 24 hours.[16]

Taking experience with adult stroke population into account, we know that treatment windows for stroke are well founded on strong scientific evi-dence: 4.5 hours for thrombolysis and/or 6 hours for mechanical thrombectomy. The implementa-tion of treatment protocols in Comprehensive Stroke Centers has achieved an improvement in quality of life for the patients, as well as a reduc-tion in costs.[17] As discussed in other chapters of this book, the treatment window has been enlarged through the use of new imaging techni-ques for mechanical thrombectomy, up to 16 or even 24 hours from the onset of symptoms of ischemic stroke.

In contrast to the scientific revolution we are witnessing in the adult population, it can hardly be believed that we know so little about diagnosis and treatment of pediatric stroke, and that we have now such scant evidence for our clinical practice.

In several ways the creation of pediatric stroke protocols has reduced diagnostic delay, always in association with increased use of MR.

According to several reports, increased suspicion and the implementation of adequate protocols have jointly achieved a reduction in the time elapsed between hospital admission and specific imaging.[18,19] On account of this striking fact, we must conclude that we must contribute to increase clinical suspicion in the daily practice of specialists and work on the implementation of protocols that bring the children earlier to emergency imaging techniques, in spite of the multiple hospital factors that work against an early diagnosis in childhood.

11.6 Neuroimaging in Pediatric Stroke

The constant advance of imaging has provided a great quantity of techniques for the assessment of the acute event and its etiopathogenesis. Computerized tomography without contrast (CT), angiotomography (ACT), magnetic resonance (MR), angioresonance (AMR) and digital subtraction angiography (DSA) all bring us closer to a correct assessment of the lesion and its etiopathogenesis, while cerebral perfusion studies allow us to establish neuronal outcome in terms of ischemic injury, and to define if the lesion can revert or not.

CT is the initial method of choice to study an adult patient if stroke is suspected, because it is the quickest and the most widespread imaging method; above all, it is most useful to rule out hemorrhage. For pediatric patients, however, this study should be limited to facilities where emergency MR cannot be done.[20] MR is the method of choice in children because it does not use ionizing radiation and therefore avoids potential adverse effects in individuals with high life expectancy. MR can also rule out other childhood conditions that may present as a stroke and cannot be diagnosed with CT, such as demyelinating diseases arising from alterations in myelin formation, and other stroke mimics.[20,21]

Contrary to popular belief relating to the usefulness of CT in ruling out brain hemorrhage, new sequences of magnetic susceptibility in MR achieve a comparable degree of sensitivity and specificity for that pathology and even achieve better results in the case of hemorrhages progressing to chronicity.[22,23] MR offers more advantages: high sensitivity and specificity for the early diagnosis of stroke (nearly 100%) and the definition of ischemic penumbra areas.[21,22]

Diffusion techniques and apparent diffusion coefficient (ADC) sequences permit prompt and early diagnosis of stroke, within minutes of onset, in fact. If perfusion MR, using gadolinium as contrast agent, is added to complete the study, the hypoperfusion zone or penumbra zone can be determined and on the basis of those data a decision on treatment can be reached.

A comparison of the images from those two techniques enables to infer the amount of salvageable parenchyma if treatment (fibrinolysis or thrombectomy) is undertaken. If the hypoperfusion zone is greater than the infarcted zone (as seen by the diffusion images), the situation is described as 'diffusion-perfusion mismatch'.

MR scan has, however, some disadvantages in comparison with CT: less equipment is available and sedation is necessary for pediatric patients in order to carry out the study.

Patients who have been diagnosed for stroke during their MR scan must have their study completed by AMR in order to rule out large-vessel occlusion. This scan, which is done without contrast, depends on arterial flow. Therefore, its sensitivity is inferior to that of methods depending on vascular filling like activated clotting time (ACT) or digital subtraction angiography (DSA).

If the initial study was a CT that ruled out hemorrhage, the study must be completed with ACT with intravenous contrast in order to rule out arterial occlusion as well.

If ACT or AMR suggests some vascular alteration, whether arterial or venous, the patient must have a DSA, this method being the gold standard for these conditions.[24,25]

DSA is the method of choice for the study of intracranial and cervical vascular pathology.[24,25] Although an invasive technique, it is very useful, especially to determine the cause of a cerebral occlusion and its location or to discover aneurysms or vascular malformations as causes for hemorrhage. On the other hand, in spite of the increasing technological improvements and the development of new techniques like CT in the angiography suite and the possibility of perfusion studies, we believe that DSA will not be substituted by these techniques when it comes to vascular assessment. The rate of complications is extremely low in DSA. When done by experts it is a safe study that can contribute very valuable data for an etiology-based diagnosis of stroke, its adequate treatment and its long-term prognosis.[25]

11.7 A Review of Modifiable Factors

11.7.1 Acute Stabilization

Stabilization is a fundamental part of care in the pediatric patient suspected of ischemic stroke. It aims at minimizing brain injury with the consequent improvement of outcome. It also helps to optimize neurological functions and by that means, to prevent recurrences.

11.7.2 Blood Pressure

The role of blood pressure variations in children cannot be extrapolated, unfortunately, to the whole of the pediatric population on account of the different trigger factors. The few studies on the relationship of BP and ischemic stroke that are to be found in scientific literature are contradictory: some cohort studies associate high blood pressure with longer hospitalizations and an increase in mortality,[26] while others rule out such possibilities.[27]

11.7.3 Temperature

When fever presents in association with stroke, it generally leads to a suspicion of concurrent sepsis or to different heart conditions or neurological diseases that are frequently associated with stroke, like endocarditis, bacterial vasculitis, etc. Fever by itself is not a risk factor that can exert influence on the outcome of ischemic stroke.

11.7.4 Glycemia

It is well-known that both hyperglycemia and hypoglycemia are harmful to brain development. There is no strong evidence, however, to support its playing the role of independent predictor of the outcome of ischemic stroke in children.

11.7.5 Oxygen Supplementation

Ischemic stroke patients are generally thought to improve their mitochondrial function with oxygen supplementation. In fact, however, nonhypoxic patients may actually do worse under oxygen because of the increased production of free radicals. Therefore, oxygen administration to patients whose oxygen levels are normal for their age is debatable.

11.7.6 Hydration

Dehydration has been associated with worse clinical outcomes in adults,[28] but there is no evidence of such a relationship in the pediatric population. There exists a clear relationship between the osmolarity increase brought about by dehydration and the increased risk of a prothrombotic state, however, and on that account prevention of dehydration should be considered in all cases of pediatric stroke.

11.7.7 Seizures

Seizures are very nearly a distinctive feature of ischemic stroke in both adult and pediatric populations. It is 18 times more frequent in children than in adults.[29] The incidence of seizures in stroke decreases with increasing age, from the newborn period onwards. Seizures may appear at onset, during the acute phase or after brain infarct has occurred. There is a clear relationship, however, between the presence of seizures at onset and after stroke. A Kaiser Permanente review demonstrated that 27% of children with stroke presenting with stroke were younger and were 5 times more likely to develop seizures during a 4-year follow-up period.[30]

Another study shows that the risk of epilepsy is 30 times greater in children with prolonged seizures during an ischemic stroke episode.[31]

The Australian Childhood Stroke Advisory Committee recommends the use of anticonvulsants in the acute phase of ischemic stroke in children with prolonged or recurrent seizures. This recommendation is included in their excellent guide for the management of stroke of childhood, with III-2, III-3 level of evidence.[16]

11.8 Treatment

11.8.1 Reperfusion Treatments

Fibrinolysis

As opposed to the situation in adults, in children the evidence in favor of fibrinolysis is lacking. Furthermore, the exact dose of fibrinolytics to be administered is unknown. Many health organizations do not authorize the use of rTPA (recombinant Tissue Plasminogen Activators) because studies demonstrating their efficacy in children are also lacking.

To extrapolate the vast available experience in adults would be a grave mistake on several accounts. Basically the causes of stroke are clearly different for both populations, and so are their clinical manifestations. On the other hand the levels of endogenous plasminogen show some variation within the pediatric population itself. The difference with adult levels is marked, childhood levels being particularly low. Inversely, activated plasminogen levels are high in children. Furthermore, there are differences in brain hemodynamics. On account of all those differences, it is to be supposed that the adequate dose for thrombolysis in brain vessels should be different for each case.

The causes of stroke are quite numerous in children; on those grounds, a correct vascular diagnosis is particularly necessary in order to define whether the disease the child is suffering from is a consequence of a thrombus and not something else, and that consideration should come well before all thought of fibrinolytics.

From 2006 onwards, the National Institute of Neurological Disorders and Stroke (NINDS) started assessing the possibility of a prospective multicentric study for the use of rTPA in children. In 2010, Thrombolysis in Pediatric Stroke TIPS emerged as a result. It was a prospective multicentric cohort dosage-finding study. Children aged 2 to 17 years were included. They were admitted if less than 4.5 hours had elapsed since onset of symptoms. An rTPA dose of 0.75 mg to 0.9–1.0 mg/kg was set. Recruiting started in October 2012, but one year later the National Institutes of Health closed the study due to lack of accrual.[32] By the end of the trial, 63% of the initial 22 centers had recruited no patients; the reasons cited were logistic and economic problems, differences in recruiting criteria and adaptation difficulties to react promptly to consent. Whatever the cause, the indisputable fact is that fibrinolysis as a treatment in children was severely affected scientifically and has not recovered since. The initial idea was that adequate dosage would be the problem, but the actual data indicate that the main problem was the lack of accrual on multiple grounds.

It could be that the need of etiological vascular diagnosis (by means of DSA, for example) in specialized centers is at the root of all this. An early clinical suspicion to direct treatment would be another important lack. The American Heart Association guidelines state that "Until there are additional published safety and efficacy data, tPA generally is not recommended for children with arterial ischaemic stroke outside a clinical trial".[33] In fact, less than 1% of the children in DeVeber's study had received thrombolytics.[34]

Mechanical Thrombectomy

In the use of mechanical thrombectomy in children the same phenomenon was observed as in fibrinolysis: it did not have the revolutionary effect it evidenced in adults with ischemic stroke. Up to the present no multicentric studies have assessed the viability of thrombectomy techniques in children, but the American Guidelines for Endovascular Treatment consider that the use of such techniques is reasonable in children younger than 18 years in whom large vessel occlusion (LVO) has been demonstrated.[35] A review of relevant literature, however, only shows case reports related to older children, chosen according to different criteria and frequently affected by heart disease. It is essential to carry out more relevant studies before giving this treatment a more important role in the management of these patients.

11.8.2 Use of Anticoagulants And Platelet Antiaggregants

As DeVeber and Kirton point out in their study, antithrombotic treatment is currently increasing, a trend that started in the last few years. About 60% of the children in their series had received either anticoagulants or AAS.[34]

As usual, pediatric studies supporting the use of therapies with high-quality evidence are few. The evidence is chrystal clear for adults, but no supporting randomized studies have been done in children. Several isolated studies, however, report on the usefulness of antiaggregants and anticoagulants in children with ischemic stroke. The use of LMWH (low-molecular -weight heparin) would seem more adequate. In some cases, clinical practice clearly shows good results; that is the case with cerebral venous thromboses, subintimal arterial dissections and cardioembolic pathology. Real evidence being unavailable, those results would provide a justification for the use of anticoagulants and platelet antiaggregants.

Corticosteroid Treatment

On scant evidence, corticosteroid treatment aims at controlling immunological response to certain pathogenic mechanisms related to ischemic stroke in children affected by varicella, enteroviruses and herpes virus.

Management of Intracranial Hypertension- Decompressive Craniectomy

About 12% of the pediatric stroke population also presents a malignant infarct caused by the occlusion of a cerebral artery.[16] Intracranial hypertension may develop if the cranial sutures are closed. Surgery in the form of decompressive craniectomy may be justified in that case.

The Australian Guidelines for the Management of Pediatric Stroke recommend the following:

Early recognition of the minority of pediatric patients with acute stroke who may develop raised intracranial pressure should prompt initial supportive care and early neurosurgical referral for consideration of decompressive craniectomy. Level of Evidence (IV).

Practice Statement:The most important indicators for raised intracranial pressure with both supra- and infratentorial infarcts are deteriorating level of consciousness and worsening of neurologic dysfunction. Due to the small space between the cranial vault and brain parenchyma children with large infarcts require close monitoring for signs and symptoms of raised intracranial pressure in the days following the stroke. Children presenting with a PedNIHSS score ≥ 8 or seizures greater than five minutes, should remain under close surveillance, as these are reported independent predictors of paediatric malignant middle cerebral artery infarction (mMCAI).

Elevated serum glucose at presentation and larger volume strokes on neuroimaging with combined involvement of cortex, white matter and basal ganglia in children older than two years are also risk factors for development of mMCAI. Level of Evidence (CBR, III-3)

Initial supportive care includes intensive neurological surveillance, 30°elevation of the head of the bed, good oxygenation, adequate hydration and maintenance of euvolaemia, nil oral intake, temperature control (avoiding hyperthermia), prevention of hypotension but toleration of mild hypertension and control of seizures.

Early neurosurgical referral is important for consideration of decompressive craniectomy and placement of intracranial pressure measuring devices. Although reliable measurement of raised intracranial pressure may be important, the placement of measuring devices or sustained medical management should not delay the more active treatment option of timely decompressive craniectomy.

Decompressive craniectomy should be considered for children with malignant ischemic MCA (or ICA) territory infarction. Level of Evidence (III, IV).[16,34]

11.9 Prognosis and Outcomes

Historically recorded mortality amounted to nearly 10%, and sequels (motor or cognitive, epilepsy) varied between 50 and 70%. Recurrence varied between 10 and 20%, the higher percentages corresponding to arteriopathy cases and patients who had not been under antithrombotic treatment.

The latest determination of mortality was 5%.[34] It is higher in newborns, but on the other hand, their recurrence risk is lower (3–5%). Focal neurological deficit amounted to 60% of newborns and 70% of older children in this series, recurrence rate being 12% and likewise related to arteriopathy and lack of antithrombotic treatment.

References

[1] Lauren A. Abstract 15: Mortality After Pediatric Arterial Ischemic Stroke: Results From the International Paediatric Stroke Study. Stroke. 2018; 49:A15

[2] Fullerton HJ, Wu YW, Zhao S, Johnston SC. Risk of stroke in children: ethnic and gender disparities. Neurology. 2003; 61 (2):189–194

[3] Lynch JK, Hirtz DG, DeVeber G, Nelson KB. Report of the National Institute of Neurological Disorders and Stroke workshop on perinatal and childhood stroke. Pediatrics. 2002; 109 (1):116–123

[4] González G, Russi ME, Crosa R. Accidente Cerebro Vascular en la infancia y la adolescencia. Ediciones Journal.2011; 1–13

[5] Fullerton HJ, Wu YW, Zhao S, Johnston SC. Risk of stroke in children: ethnic and gender disparities. Neurology. 2003; 61 (2):189–194

[6] Ong BY, Ellison PH, Browning C. Intrauterine stroke in the neonate. Arch Neurol. 1983; 40(1):55–56

[7] Golomb MR, MacGregor DL, Domi T, et al. Presumed pre- or perinatal arterial ischemic stroke: risk factors and outcomes. Ann Neurol. 2001; 50(2):163–168

[8] Lasjaunias P, Ter Brugge KG, Berenstein A. Clinical and Interventional Aspects in Children. Surgical Neuro-angiography. Vol 3. Arterial Ischemic Stroke. Springer-Verlag Berlin Heidelberg; 2006:851–908

[9] Sofronas M, Ichord RN, Fullerton HJ, et al. Pediatric stroke initiatives and preliminary studies: What is known and what is needed? Pediatr Neurol. 2006; 34(6):439–445

[10] Hills NK, Johnston SC, Sidney S, Zielinski BA, Fullerton HJ. Recent trauma and acute infection as risk factors for childhood arterial ischemic stroke. Ann Neurol. 2012; 72(6):850–858

[11] Fox CK, Hills NK, Vinson DR, et al. Population-based study of ischemic stroke risk after trauma in children and young adults. Neurology. 2017; 89(23):2310–2316

[12] Russi ME, González G, Crosa R, et al. [Dissections of craniocervical arteries in the paediatric age: a pathology that is emerging or under-diagnosed?]. Rev Neurol. 2010; 50(5): 257–264

[13] Sébire G, Tabarki B, Saunders DE, et al. Cerebral venous sinus thrombosis in children: risk factors, presentation, diagnosis and outcome. Brain. 2005; 128(Pt 3):477–489

[14] Ichord RN, Bastian R, Abraham L, et al. Interrater reliability of the Pediatric National Institutes of Health Stroke Scale (PedNIHSS) in a multicenter study. Stroke. 2011; 42 (3):613–617

[15] Rafay MF, Pontigon AM, Chiang J, et al. Delay to diagnosis in acute pediatric arterial ischemic stroke. Stroke. 2009; 40(1): 58–64

[16] Australian Childhood Stroke Advisory Committee. Guideline for the diagnosis and acute management of childhood stroke. available from: https://www.mcri.edu.au/sites/default/files/media/stroke_guidelines.pdf– 2017

[17] Stroke Foundation. National Stroke Audit of Acute Services 2015. Available from: https://informme.org.au. Accessed March 2017

[18] Ladner TR, Mahdi J, Gindville MC, et al. Pediatric Acute Stroke Protocol Activation in a Children's Hospital Emergency Department. Stroke. 2015; 46(8):2328–2331

[19] DeLaroche AM, Sivaswamy L, Farooqi A, Kannikeswaran N. Pediatric Stroke Clinical Pathway Improves the Time to Diagnosis in an Emergency Department. Pediatr Neurol. 2016; 65:39–44

[20] Mirsky DM, Beslow LA, Amlie-Lefond C, et al. International Paediatric Stroke Study Neuroimaging Consortium and the Paediatric Stroke Neuroimaging Consortium. Pathways for Neuroimaging of Childhood Stroke. Pediatr Neurol. 2017; 69: 11–23

[21] Mathews JD, Forsythe AV, Brady Z, et al. Cancer risk in 680,000 people exposed to computed tomography scans in childhood or adolescence: data linkage study of 11 million Australians. BMJ. 2013; 346:f2360

[22] Mitomi M, Kimura K, Aoki J, Iguchi Y. Comparison of CT and DWI findings in ischemic stroke patients within 3 hours of onset. J Stroke Cerebrovasc Dis. 2014; 23(1):37–42

[23] Liu AC, Segaren N, Cox TS, et al. Is there a role for magnetic resonance imaging in the evaluation of non-traumatic intra-parenchymal haemorrhage in children? Pediatr Radiol. 2006; 36(9):940–946

[24] Husson B, Lasjaunias P. Radiological approach to disorders of arterial brain vessels associated with childhood arterial stroke-a comparison between MRA and contrast angiography. Pediatr Radiol. 2004; 34(1):10–15

[25] Burger IM, Murphy KJ, Jordan LC, Tamargo RJ, Gailloud P. Safety of cerebral digital subtraction angiography in children: complication rate analysis in 241 consecutive diagnostic angiograms. Stroke. 2006; 37(10):2535–2539

[26] Adil MM, Beslow LA, Qureshi AI, Malik AA, Jordan LC. Hypertension is Associated With Increased Mortality in Children Hospitalized With Arterial Ischemic Stroke. Pediatr Neurol. 2016; 56:25–29

[27] Grelli KN, Gindville MC, Walker CH, Jordan LC. Association of Blood Pressure, Blood Glucose, and Temperature With Neurological Outcome After Childhood Stroke. JAMA Neurol. 2016; 73(7):829–835

[28] Liu CH, Lin SC, Lin JR, et al. Dehydration is an independent predictor of discharge outcome and admission cost in acute ischaemic stroke. Eur J Neurol. 2014; 21(9):1184–1191

[29] Chadehumbe MA, Khatri P, Khoury JC, et al. Seizures are common in the acute setting of childhood stroke: a population-based study. J Child Neurol. 2009; 24(1):9–12

[30] Fox CK, Glass HC, Sidney S, Lowenstein DH, Fullerton HJ. Acute seizures predict epilepsy after childhood stroke. Ann Neurol. 2013; 74(2):249–256

[31] Fox CK, Mackay MT, Dowling MM, et al. Prolonged or recurrent acute seizures after pediatric arterial ischemic stroke are associated with increasing epilepsy risk. Dev Med Child Neurol. 2016

[32] Rivkin MJ, deVeber G, Ichord RN, et al. Thrombolysis in pediatric stroke study. Stroke. 2015; 46(3):880–885

[33] Roach ES, Golomb MR, Adams R, et al. American Heart Association Stroke Council, Council on Cardiovascular Disease in the Young. Management of stroke in infants and children: a scientific statement from a Special Writing Group of the American Heart Association Stroke Council and the Council on Cardiovascular Disease in the Young. Stroke. 2008; 39(9): 2644–2691

[34] deVeber GA, Kirton A, Booth FA, et al. Epidemiology and Outcomes of Arterial Ischemic Stroke in Children: The Canadian Pediatric Ischemic Stroke Registry. Pediatr Neurol. 2017; 69: 58–70

[35] Powers WJ, Derdeyn CP, Biller J, et al. American Heart Association Stroke Council. 2015 American Heart Association/American Stroke Association Focused Update of the 2013 Guidelines for the Early Management of Patients With Acute Ischemic Stroke Regarding Endovascular Treatment: A Guideline for Healthcare Professionals From the American Heart Association/American Stroke Association. Stroke. 2015; 46 (10):3020–3035

12 The Future in Ischemic Stroke: New Techniques

Christopher Hilditch, Patrick Nicholson, Adam A. Dmytriw and Vitor Mendes Pereira

Abstract

Workflow optimization is without a doubt the next major hurdle for stroke intervention in an era where selection and endovascular tools have been honed. Specific areas of intense work include prehospital detection and rapid transfer to centers capable of comprehensive treatment as well as early neuroprotection. Thereafter, modification of approach based on individualized factors such as premorbid condition, anatomy, and clot composition have become a major focus. As endovascular technologies improve, the window for meaningful intervention has markedly increased. With this comes a need to identify clinical and imaging parameters which may as better indicators of candidacy than mere time post-ictus. Here we discuss some of the major current and upcoming milestones following the era of the major trials and meta-analyses.

Keywords: workflow, neuroprotection, technology, access, personalization

12.1 Prehospital Detection Of Stroke

The current tenet of stroke care is to identify the patient suffering from an acute ischemic stroke (AIS) as quickly and efficiently as possible, and then to transport them to the nearest stroke center for imaging and initial acute medical care. Patients with a confirmed large vessel occlusion (LVO) on imaging are then transported if necessary to a hospital with endovascular stroke treatment (EVT) capabilities. There is still much uncertainty regarding the optimal pathway for these patients. Should they be directly transferred to a comprehensive stroke center with mechanical thrombectomy capabilities, bypassing the often nearer primary stroke center? Or should they be imaged and assessed locally, therefore transferring only the candidates that are amenable to EVT to the comprehensive stroke center? If so, what about the time lost in assessment at the primary center? We can learn some lessons from the trauma bypass and ST Elevation Myocardial Infarction (STEMI) bypass systems employed by our colleagues in other specialties. In addition, one randomized controlled trial will randomize patients in Catalonia, Spain to these various pathways in an effort to ascertain the one that will provide the best clinical outcomes. This is the RACECAT study (ClinicalTrials.gov Identifier: NCT02795962)[1] which as of the date of this writing is currently recruiting, and the stroke community awaits the results of this with some interest. In addition, there are a number of points at which these prehospital processes can be improved, and work is ongoing in these areas.

12.2 Stroke Scales

The use of stroke scales by paramedics/emergency medical technicians to identify patients at high likelihood of having an LVO is not a new concept. Several such stroke scores exist, including the Rapid Arterial Occlusion Evaluation (RACE), Cincinnati Prehospital Stroke Scale (CPSS), Field Assessment Stroke Triage For Emergency Destination (FAST-ED), Vision Aphasia Neglect (VAN), Los Angeles Motor Scale (LAMS), and Prehospital Acute Stroke Severity (PASS) scale. No universally accepted score exists, however, and there is no universally accepted cutoff for each score. The National Institute of Health Stroke Scale (NIHSS), meanwhile, was initially designed for use as a research tool and is not best suited for use in the prehospital setting. Any proposed score will need to avoid underdiagnosing patients (and thereby missing potentially eligible EVT candidates, while avoiding overdiagnosis (in order to prevent "flooding" the receiving hospital with stroke mimics and other non-EVT candidates). In addition, each prehospital care provider will need to be trained in the use of the agreed stroke scale, as well as educated in the need for rapid transfer of these eligible patients to an EVT center. Finally, any of these scoring systems as well as any future scoring systems will need to be externally validated in potential EVT-eligible AIS patients. They will also need to prove that they can help improve clinical outcomes in getting patients to the comprehensive stroke centers more quickly.

12.3 Prehospital Stroke Detection Devices

Several groups are working on improving the prehospital detection of AIS patients. One focus is on the use of biomarkers, as measured by point-of-care (POC) assays. These are analogous to the pre-hospital use of troponin measurement in cardiac patients and if adopted would have the advantage of being relatively cheap and easy to replicate in other jurisdictions. Many different biomarkers have been studied for this purpose, but none has proven particularly efficacious. Potential reasons include the effect of the cerebral blood-brain barrier (BBB) in limiting biomarker release into the peripheral circulation, as well as the fact that most research to date has focused on AIS patients after they have been admitted, and there is very little research on the detection of these biomarkers early in the patient's stroke. Another focus is in the use of prehospital detection devices, most of which primarily use transcranial Doppler ultrasound (e.g., the Lucid M1 Transcranial Doppler System [Neural Analytics] and SONAS System [BURL Concepts]). These comprise a helmet that contains multiple transducers/sensors and can be placed over the patient's head. The purpose of such helmet devices would ideally be to quantity disparity in cerebral blood flow in a semi-automated fashion. Other devices utilize noninvasive cerebral oximetry with similar aims.[2] To date, no such system has gained widespread use; they have only been used in small trials and all require large-scale validation in an unselected cohort of AIS patients (▶ Fig. 12.1).

A third focus which has gained more widespread popularity is the use of mobile stroke units (MSUs), first popularized in Germany in the early 2000s. These comprise of a CT scanner mounted in the ambulance, which can provide onsite imaging in terms of both noncontrast CT brain scans (to exclude hemorrhage and evaluate the degree of infarction) and even CT angiography (to confirm LVO), with physician analysis and support via telemedicine. While some studies have shown that the use of such MSUs can decrease the time to tPA in

AIS patients[3] no study to date has proven that the use of these units results in improved clinical outcome for patients. In addition, given the sizeable financial outlay of these units (both in terms of upfront costs and ongoing costs), future studies will need to prove the cost-effectiveness of this approach before they can gain widespread clinical use.

12.4 Transfers Direct To Angiosuite

The possibility of transferring AIS patients directly from the ambulance onto the neuro-angiography suite table is an ambitious but potential patient pathway solution. This may be for interhospital transfers or for patients who have been identified as having a high likelihood of LVO in the prehospital setting by using some of the previously described methods. Much work has been published previously on various simple but effective workflow steps that, when implemented, can save valuable minutes off the door-to-puncture time.[4] These include prenotification for all-stroke team members, preregistration of the patient before arrival, and so on. These all play a role in the direct-to-angio model, but the real rate-limiting step for this approach is the on-table imaging. In order to fully bypass the emergency department and its multislice CT/CTA/CTP capabilities, the angiosuite must be able to offer comparable imaging. Thankfully, recent research has allowed us to take steps in this direction. The acquisition of CTA images on the angio table is relatively straightforward.[5] Meanwhile the addition of flat panel detectors to modern angiosuites (FD-CT) has enabled an improvement in image quality so that noncontrast images of the brain parenchyma—essential for grading the degree of established infarction— rival those obtained on traditional CT scanners. This is a

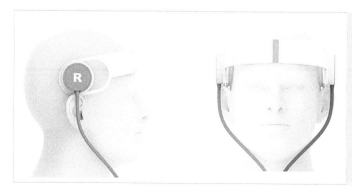

Fig. 12.1 SONAS device (BURL Concepts).

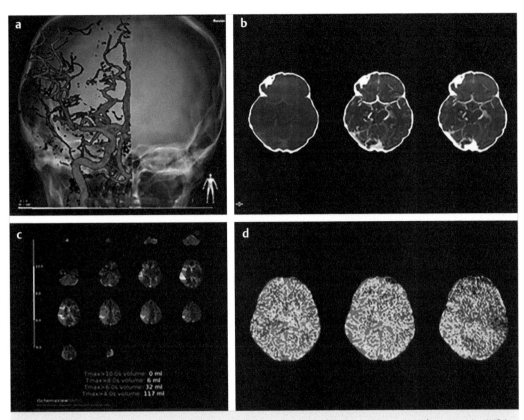

Fig. 12.2 CTA and CT perfusion imaging obtained from the angiosuite.**(a, b)** CTA reconstructions demonstrating LVO in the right M1. **(c)** RAPID CT perfusion analysis demonstrates prolonged mean transit time (MTT) in the right MCA territory. **(d)** Flat panel CT perfusion images demonstrate delayed perfusion (via collaterals) in the affected territory.

truly exciting step, which will enable us to offer a "one-stop" imaging pathway for our AIS patients (▶ Fig. 12.2).

12.5 Neuroprotective Agents in Acute Stroke

The use of neuroprotective agents for AIS as adjuvant therapy for patients receiving intravenous thrombolysis (IVT) has shown promise in preclinical models, but this has so far failed to translate into clinical success.[6] The target for these agents is to reduce neuronal death within the ischemic penumbra adjacent to already infarcted brain tissue by promoting neuronal recovery and plasticity.[7] Currently there are numerous agents undergoing preclinical evaluation, with some demonstrating promise.

Excitotoxicity is a key mediator in the process of neuronal death during an ischemic stroke. Depolarization resulting from adenosine triphosphate (ATP) depletion causes failure to maintain membrane potentials in the neuron. Glutamate is released from the neurons, and this overwhelms the synaptic connections between neurons with excessive activation of ionotropic glutamatergic receptors (e.g., N-methyl-D-aspartate [NMDA] receptor). Eventually, there is uncontrolled calcium entry into the cell bodies, causing cell death. Furthermore, excited neurons will also release their neurotransmitter stores, leading to propagating waves of neuronal activity followed by electrical silencing, so-called peri-infarct depolarization, which exacerbates the severity of ischemic damage.[6,8] Targeting this mechanism of brain damage via excitotoxicity has been evaluated in clinical trials using NMDA antagonists, but these have failed to demonstrate benefits in patients. More recently, more specific targets in this pathway of neuronal death are being evaluated, rather than blanket blockade of NMDA receptors.

One such example is NA-1, which is a peptide that disrupts interactions between NMDA receptor subunits and more specifically uncouples the neuronal nitric oxide synthase (nNOS) enzyme from glutamate receptor activation, resulting in less production of nitric oxide (NO), which is damaging to neurons in an acute infarction. A previous phase II clinical trial evaluating NA-1 administered to patients undergoing endovascular repair of cerebral aneurysms demonstrated positive findings, with reduction of cerebral infarcts detected on MRI in patients receiving the agent.[9] A larger randomized controlled trial is underway evaluating the efficacy and safety of intravenous NA-1 in patients undergoing EVT.[10]

Approaches to target other key features of ischemia-mediated brain damage have been investigated. These include disruption of the generation of free radicals as well as modulating the immune responses to an ischemically damaged brain. Hypothermia can reduce oxygen demand in the ischemic brain and also reduce enzyme degradation, cellular acidosis and neuronal neurotransmitter uptake. Studies have demonstrated potential improvement of neurologic outcomes with cooling in patients with acute stroke.[7] Multiple other novel approaches have been and are being investigated as potential methods of neuroprotection, including administration of hyperbaric oxygen, stem cell therapy, anti-epileptic drugs, and even caffeine and alcohol. A summary table of some key neuroprotective agents and strategies under investigation is provided in ▶ Table 12.1.

Neuroprotection is clearly a potential means of improving outcomes in ischemic stroke, but few studies have as yet demonstrated clear clinical benefits. Future directions for investigation of these strategies will be primarily focused on how they can be delivered to patients at the optimal time point of their acute management. This may be prehospital administration, as an adjunct in patients undergoing EVT or intra-arterial delivery.[16]

12.6 Current Status of Aspiration vs. Stent Retrievers and Clot Composition

Following the publication of six randomized controlled trials for EVT in acute stroke, its benefit over standard medical therapy alone is beyond question.[17] Retrievable stents were the primary endovascular technique used in these trials. Subsequently, supple large-bore aspiration catheters became more widely available, and the question has been raised as to which technique results in faster and more reliable large vessel recanalization safely.

A direct first pass technique (ADAPT) involves direct aspiration as a first-line method, followed by adding a stent retriever (with adjunct aspiration) as a second pass if required. The ASTER randomized controlled trial[18] has been recently published which compared the efficacy and adverse events of first-line thrombectomy using direct aspiration vs. the first-line use of stent

Table 12.1 Key neuroprotective agents and strategies under investigation

Neuroprotective agent/ strategy	Mechanism	Results	Reference
NA-1	Regulation and expression of NMDA channels	Imaging benefit in patients receiving IV NA-1 following cerebral endovascular procedures	Hill, 2012[7]
Ginsenoside	Calcium channel blocker	Better NIHSS at 15 days	Liu, 2009[11]
Natalizumab	Immune modulating monoclonal antibody	Better mRS at 90 days in treated patients	Elkins, 2017[12]
Fingolimod	Immune modulator	Better mRS and NIHSS at 90 days in treated patients	Zhu, 2015[13]
Hypothermia	Brain cooling	Awaited	iCOOL2 (NCT01584167)[14]
Remote ischemic preconditioning (RIPC)	Inducing ischemia in a different tissue/organ to promote ischemic tolerance in the brain	Awaited	Pico, 2016[15]

retrievers. The primary outcome was the percentage of successful recanalization, define as modified Thrombolysis in Cerebral Infarction (mTICI) score 2b or better. Secondary outcomes included time from arterial puncture to recanalization and modified Rankin Score (mRS) at 90 days, including an mRS shift analysis. Three hundred eighty-one patients were randomized, with 192 receiving first pass aspiration and 189 receiving first pass stent retriever thrombectomy. Patients received three attempts of their assigned technique (direct aspiration alone or stent retriever alone). If this did not result in mTICI 2b/3, then operators switched to a different "rescue therapy"; this was decided at their discretion and included aspiration, stent retriever, stent retriever with aspiration, and angioplasty with or without stenting. No statistical difference was recorded in the percentage of mTICI 2b/3 recanalization rates achieved between the two groups, nor was there any difference in time to revascularization, mRS at 90 days or adverse events between the two groups. No statistical difference in the number of attempts using the assigned technique was recorded.

Direct aspiration and stent retriever thrombectomy appear to be equivalent when used as first-pass methods for EVT. The choice of EVT method is clearly influenced by operator experience. Anecdotally, many operators may choose either aspiration or a stent retriever based on the site of the occlusion. The first-choice aspiration catheters for proximal occlusions in the M1 or M2 segments of the middle cerebral artery are generally in the 6- and 5-French size category. More distal occlusions in M2 or M3 branches may be more amenable to recanalization using a stent retriever than an aspiration catheter, which may be too large to reach small distal intracranial vessels. Interestingly, the ASTER trial[18] results show that there were more patients with M2 occlusion in the direct aspiration group than the stent retriever group. A recent study has demonstrated safe and effective recanalization of distal small M2 and M3 middle cerebral artery branches using a smaller-bore aspiration catheter measuring 3.8-French.[19] Smaller stents are also available, and studies have demonstrated safety and efficacy when these stents are used to reopen smaller more fragile distal vessels.[20] Occlusions involving the A2 segment of the anterior cerebral artery are particularly challenging; more research regarding the safety of the use of aspiration catheters and stent retrievers in this artery is required.

The effectiveness of EVT and IVT may vary with clot composition, and different EVT methods may be more effective in retrieving different types of clots than others. Clot composition may vary depending on the aetiology of the embolism, and this may be detectable using imaging. Indeed, studies have demonstrated that not all cerebral clots are the same; however, the literature is conflicting. Boeckh-Behrens et al demonstrated that clots originating from cardiac sources contained a higher proportion of fibrin and platelets than red blood cells compared to noncardioembolic stroke.[21] Other studies have found different results. Kim et al reported the converse, in that strokes due to cardioembolism contained a higher proportion of red blood cells and less fibrin compared to strokes from large artery atherosclerosis such as those due to internal carotid artery atheromatous plaque rupture.[22] Clot composition may be predicted prior to EVT using MR imaging modalities such as gradient echo sequences to look for susceptibility artefact due to iron in red blood cell-rich clots.[22]

Fibrin-rich clots are often deemed more difficult to extract from a cerebral blood vessel, requiring a greater number of passes than thrombi rich in red blood cells.[23] Concomitant medical therapy may also alter clot composition in patients presenting with acute stroke; indeed, the use of IVT has been reported to be associated with fibrinolytic effects on fibrin-rich clots, which may make the clot more retrievable.[24] Research involving clot analogues and models that replicate the cerebral circulation is being undertaken to identify strategies to tailor recanalization methods to individual patients depending on their stroke etiology and clot composition.[23]

12.7 Balloon Guide Catheters

The use of balloon guide catheters during EVT has been shown to be associated with better reperfusion rates and improved clinical outcomes.[25] This result is due to the promotion of flow arrest and even flow reversal, which theoretically maximizes clot retrieval and minimizes distal embolization of clot fragments, which can be mobilized during EVT. Remote aspiration using balloon guide catheters may result in fewer instances of distal emboli due to clot fragmentation, since the devices used for thrombectomy do not come into contact with the clot itself. Currently, there is a lack of published literature on this topic; however, a recent case series[26] demonstrated that successful and complete recanalization of distal internal carotid artery occlusions can be achieved using remote aspiration through a balloon guide catheter.

12.8 Expanding the Therapeutic Window for EVT in Acute Stroke

The previous randomized controlled trials that demonstrated EVT superiority over standard medical therapy did so when EVT was performed within 6 hours of stroke onset.[27] New trials have recently been published suggesting that EVT can be performed between 6 and 24 hours after stroke onset. The DAWN trial[27] enrolled patients with occlusion of the intracranial internal carotid artery or the proximal middle cerebral artery who had been last seen well between 6 and 24 hours prior and demonstrated a mismatch between clinical symptoms and infarct core. Patients were randomly assigned to thrombectomy plus standard medical care or to standard medical care alone. The primary endpoint was mean score on the utility-weighted mRS (modified Rankin Scale) at 90 days, and secondary endpoints included early improvement of NIHSS scores, mortality, median infarct size, and rate of revascularization. Enrollment was stopped prematurely following the results of a prespecified interim analysis. The trial subdivided patients into three groups: group A were patients older than 80 years who had an NIHSS score of greater than or equal to 10 and an infarct volume of less than 21 mL (calculated by CT/MRI perfusion); group B were younger than 80 with an NIHSS score of greater than or equal to 10 and an infarct core of less than 31 mL; group C were also younger than 80 but had a more severe stroke, with an NIHSS of greater than or equal to 20 and an infarct volume of 31–51 mL. The interim analysis demonstrated clear benefit of EVT in all groups. The rate of 90-day functional independence in the patients receiving EVT was 49% compared to 13% in patients receiving medical therapy alone. All secondary outcomes favored thrombectomy.

The DEFUSE 3 trial[28] similarly investigated patients presenting late with acute stroke. Patients in this trial were last known well between 6 and 16 hours prior and demonstrated remaining ischemic brain tissue yet to be infarcted. Patients had proximal middle cerebral artery (MCA) or internal carotid artery (ICA) occlusion and an infarct volume of less than 70 mL (assessed using CT perfusion). This trial, like DAWN, was terminated early

after an interim analysis and demonstrated a clear favorable shift in 90-day mRS in the patients receiving EVT compared to those who did not. A higher percentage of patients in the EVT group achieved functional independence, and the 90-day mortality rate was significantly higher in patients who did not undergo EVT. There were no significant differences in symptomatic intracranial hemorrhages between the groups.

These trials have resulted in a change to the American Heart Association/American Stroke Association guidelines in 2018.[29] EVT now has level-1 evidence for patients with large cerebral vessel occlusions who were last seen well up to 24 hours prior.

12.9 Alternative Access for EVT

The most common route of vascular access for cerebral interventional procedures is via the common femoral artery. Strokes tend to occur in older patients or patients with hypertension. Such patients commonly have elongated and tortuous vascular anatomy as a result of their hypertension or aging. Such tortuosity, especially in the aortic arch, can make access to the cerebral vessels more difficult, if not impossible. Alternative routes are possible, such as via the radial artery or via direct common carotid artery puncture. The left common carotid artery and the right vertebral artery can be particularly difficult vessels to catheterize from a femoral approach. Radial access for cardiac coronary endovascular procedures is very well established, but not so for cerebral procedures. Several studies have demonstrated that the radial approach is feasible and safe when performing cerebral angiography, and this mode of access can be a useful tool when encountering difficult aortic arches during EVT for acute stroke. The safety of direct carotid puncture in EVT for acute stroke is not established but has been described and is feasible.[30]

12.10 Summary

The advent of EVT for AIS has changed the landscape of stroke care in the 21st century, but there are many challenges, and unanswered questions remain. Optimizing patient selection, minimizing time from onset to treatment, and choosing the most effective treatment strategy with or without pharmaceutical adjuncts for each patient are among the key future directions in this rapidly-evolving field.

References

[1] Ribo M, Abilleira S, Perez de la Ossa N. Direct Transfer to an Endovascular Center Compared to Transfer to the Closest Stroke Center in Acute Stroke Patients With Suspected Large Vessel Occlusion (RACECAT).https://clinicaltrials.Gov/ct2/show/nct02795962.

[2] Flint AC, Bhandari SG, Cullen SP, et al. Detection of Anterior Circulation Large Artery Occlusion in Ischemic Stroke Using Noninvasive Cerebral Oximetry. Stroke. 2018; 49(2):458–460

[3] Kunz A, Ebinger M, Geisler F, et al. Functional outcomes of pre-hospital thrombolysis in a mobile stroke treatment unit compared with conventional care: an observational registry study. Lancet Neurol. 2016; 15(10):1035–1043

[4] Zerna C, Assis Z, d'Esterre CD, Menon BK, Goyal M. Imaging, Intervention, and Workflow in Acute Ischemic Stroke: The Calgary Approach. AJNR Am J Neuroradiol. 2016; 37(6):978–984

[5] Struffert T, Deuerling-Zheng Y, Kloska S, et al. Dynamic Angiography and Perfusion Imaging Using Flat Detector CT in the Angiography Suite: A Pilot Study in Patients with Acute Middle Cerebral Artery Occlusions. AJNR Am J Neuroradiol. 2015; 36(10):1964–1970

[6] Neuhaus AA, Couch Y, Hadley G, Buchan AM. Neuroprotection in stroke: the importance of collaboration and reproducibility. Brain. 2017; 140(8):2079–2092

[7] Rajah GB, Ding Y. Experimental neuroprotection in ischemic stroke: a concise review. Neurosurg Focus. 2017; 42(4):E2

[8] Dreier JP. The role of spreading depression, spreading depolarization and spreading ischemia in neurological disease. Nat Med. 2011; 17(4):439–447

[9] Hill MD, Martin RH, Mikulis D, et al. ENACT trial investigators. Safety and efficacy of NA-1 in patients with iatrogenic stroke after endovascular aneurysm repair (ENACT): a phase 2, randomized, double-blind, placebo-controlled trial. Lancet Neurol. 2012; 11(11):942–950

[10] Tymianski, M. Combining neuroprotection with endovascular treatment of acute stroke: is there hope? Stroke 2017; 48:17001705

[11] Liu X, Xia J, Wang L, et al. Efficacy and safety of ginsenoside-Rd for acute ischaemic stroke: a randomized, double-blind, placebo-controlled, phase II multicenter trial. Eur J Neurol. 2009; 16(5):569–575

[12] Elkins J, Veltkamp R, Montaner J, et al. Safety and efficacy of natalizumab in patients with acute ischaemic stroke (ACTION): a randomized, placebo-controlled, double-blind phase 2 trial. Lancet Neurol. 2017; 16(3):217–226

[13] Zhu Z, Fu Y, Tian D, et al. Combination of the Immune Modulator Fingolimod With Alteplase in Acute Ischemic Stroke: A Pilot Trial. Circulation. 2015; 132(12):1104–1112

[14] Poli S, Purrucker J, Priglinger M, Ebner M, Sykora M, Diedler J, et al. Rapid Induction of COOLing in Stroke Patients (iCOOL1): A randomised pilot study comparing cold infusions with nasopharyngeal cooling. Crit Care. 2014;18:582.

[15] Pico F, Rosso C, Meseguer E, et al. A multicenter, randomized trial on neuroprotection with remote ischemic per-conditioning during acute ischemic stroke: the REmote iSchemic Conditioning in acUtE BRAin INfarction study protocol. Int J Stroke. 2016; 11(8):938–943

[16] Babadjouni RM, Radwanski RE, Walcott BP, et al. Neuroprotective strategies following intraparenchymal hemorrhage. J Neurointerv Surg. 2017; 9(12):1202–1207

[17] Goyal M, Menon BK, van Zwam WH, et al. HERMES collaborators. Endovascular thrombectomy after large-vessel ischaemic stroke: a meta-analysis of individual patient data from five randomized trials. Lancet. 2016; 387 (10029):1723–1731

[18] Lapergue B, Blanc R, Gory B, et al. ASTER Trial Investigators. Effect of endovascular contact aspiration vs stent retriever on revascularization in patients with acute ischemic stroke and large vessel occlusion: The ASTER randomized clinical trial. JAMA. 2017; 318(5):443–452

[19] Altenbernd J, Kuhnt O, Hennigs S, Hilker R, Loehr C. Frontline ADAPT therapy to treat patients with symptomatic M2 and M3 occlusions in acute ischemic stroke: initial experience with the Penumbra ACE and 3MAX reperfusion system. J Neurointerv Surg. 2017; •••:013233

[20] Kühn AL, Wakhloo AK, Lozano JD, et al. Two-year single-center experience with the 'Baby Trevo' stent retriever for mechanical thrombectomy in acute ischemic stroke. J Neurointerv Surg. 2017; 9(6):541–546

[21] Boeckh-Behrens T, Kleine JF, Zimmer C, et al. Thrombus histology suggests cardioembolic cause in cryptogenic stroke. Stroke. 2016; 47(7):1864–1871

[22] Kim SK, Yoon W, Kim TS, Kim HS, Heo TW, Park MS. Histologic analysis of retrieved clots in acute ischemic stroke: Correlation with stroke etiology and gradient-echo MRI. AJNR Am J Neuroradiol. 2015; 36(9):1756–1762

[23] Fennell VS, Setlur Nagesh SV, Meess KM, et al. What to do about fibrin rich 'tough clots'? Comparing the Solitaire stent retriever with a novel geometric clot extractor in an in vitro stroke model. J Neurointerv Surg. 2018; 10(9):907–910

[24] Krajíčková D, et al. Fibrin Clot Architecture in Acute Ischemic Stroke Treated With Mechanical Thrombectomy With Stent-Retrievers-Cohort Study. Circ J. 2017

[25] Brinjikji W, et al. Impact of balloon guide catheter on technical and clinical outcomes: a systematic review and meta-analysis. J Neurointerv Surg. 2017; •••:013179

[26] Haussen DC, Bouslama M, Grossberg JA, Nogueira RG. Remote aspiration thrombectomy in large vessel acute ischemic stroke. J Neurointerv Surg. 2017; 9(3):250–252

[27] Nogueira RG, Jadhav AP, Haussen DC, et al. DAWN Trial Investigators. Thrombectomy 6 to 24 Hours after Stroke with a Mismatch between Deficit and Infarct. N Engl J Med. 2018; 378(1):11–21

[28] Albers GW, Marks MP, Kemp S, et al. DEFUSE 3 Investigators. Thrombectomy for Stroke at 6 to 16 Hours with Selection by Perfusion Imaging. N Engl J Med. 2018; 378(8):708–718

[29] Powers WJ, Rabinstein AA, Ackerson T, et al. American Heart Association Stroke Council. 2018 Guidelines for the Early Management of Patients With Acute Ischemic Stroke: A Guideline for Healthcare Professionals From the American Heart Association/American Stroke Association. Stroke. 2018; 49 (3):e46–e110

[30] Mokin M, Snyder KV, Levy EI, Hopkins LN, Siddiqui AH. Direct carotid artery puncture access for endovascular treatment of acute ischemic stroke: technical aspects, advantages, and limitations. J Neurointerv Surg. 2015; 7(2):108–113

Index

Note: Page numbers set **bold** or *italic* indicate headings or figures, respectively.